Phar[...]

Richa[...]

Program Director
Department of Emergency Medicine
The University of Alabama at Birmingham
University of Alabama School of Medicine/Huntsville
    Program
Huntsville, Alabama

F. A. DAVIS COMPANY • Philadelphia

Publisher: Jean-François Vilain
Acquisitions Editor: Lynn Borders Caldwell
Production Editor: Jessica Howie Martin
Cover Designer: Steven Ross Morrone

Printed in the United States of America
8 9 10 XXX 05

For more information, contact Delmar, 3 Columbia Circle, PO Box 15015, Albany, NY 12212-0515; or find us on the World Wide Web at http://www.delmar.com

Library of Congress Cataloging-in-Publication Data
Beck, Richard K., 1947-
        Pharmacology field reference guide/Richard K. Beck.
            p. cm.
        Includes bibliographical references and index.
        ISBN 0-8036-0133-6
        1. Drugs—Handbooks, manuals, etc. 2. Emergency medicine—
Handbooks, manuals, etc. 3. Nursing—Handbooks, manuals, etc.
I. Title.
        [DNLM: 1. Emergencies—handbooks. 2. Drug Therapy—handbooks.
WB 39 B393p; 1996]
RM301.12.B43 1996
616.02'5—dc20   95-50500
DNLM/DLC for Library of Congress   CIP

How to Use This Field Guide

The uses of this field reference guide are many. Paramedics, paramedical students, and nurses will find this text useful at school, at clinical rotation sites, during field internships, or in any emergency-care setting. Although compact, this reference contains pertinent information on the 73 drugs most commonly administered by paramedics, and its small size makes it useful when carrying a larger text is not feasible or convenient.

In the hospital or emergency setting, for example, this handy reference guide can fit in a lab coat pocket or be stored in the ambulance or helicopter, available when needed.

The guide is divided into three sections: adult, pediatric, and general. Because most patients encountered by the paramedic are adults, this section appears first. American Heart Association treatment algorithms are included for easy reference. Medications are listed in alphabetical order by generic name so that the paramedic can locate them rapidly.

Generally, paramedics find treating children especially stressful; therefore, more reference information pertaining to children is included to help the reader. For example, included are a table for calculating pediatric drug concentrations and infusion rates, guidelines for ET tube and suction catheter size, and a section on treatment steps for newborn resuscitation. This section is an easy guide for quick reference when treatment of a child is required.

General information has been included because many times the paramedic may need a variety of general information. For example, he or she may need to know laboratory values or rules for identification of ECGs. Or, while at the emergency scene, the paramedic may need to reference the patient's prescription medications.

Acknowledgments

The author would like to thank the following reviewers for their helpful suggestions:

Margorie Bowers, EdD, RN, NREMT-P, Associate Professor, Indian River Community College, Fort Pierce, Florida

Kenneth D. Cross, RN, BS, NREMT-P, Paramedic Coordinator, University of South Alabama, Mobile, Alabama

Terry DeVito, RN, BS, EMT-P, CEN, Coordinator, Paramedic Program, Capital Community Technical College, Hartford, Connecticut

Gary G. Ferguson, PhD, Associate Professor of Pharmacology, Northeast Louisiana University (Retired), Monroe, Louisiana

Gregg S. Margolis, BS, EMT-P, Associate Director of Education, Center for Emergency Medicine, Pittsburgh, Pennsylvania

Thomas E. Platt, NREMT-P, Coordinator—EMS Education, Center for Emergency Medicine, Pittsburgh, Pennsylvania

Patricia L. Tritt, RN, MA, System Director, EMS and Trauma, Health OWE, Denver, Colorado

Contents

Emergency Phone Numbers

Unit #: _____________   Name: _____________________________________

Medical resource hospital _______________________________________

Trauma resource hospital _______________________________________

Children's hospital _______________________________________

Burn center _______________________________________

Air medical transport _______________________________________

Chemtrec 1-800-424-9300

Poison control center _______________________________________

911 communications center _______________________________________

Local EMS office _______________________________________

State EMS office _______________________________________

Health department _______________________________________

Medical examiner _______________________________________

CISD team _______________________________________

_____________________ Hospital _______________________________

_____________________ Hospital _______________________________

_____________________ Hospital _______________________________

Other _______________________________________

Other _______________________________________

Other _______________________________________

PART I: ADULTS

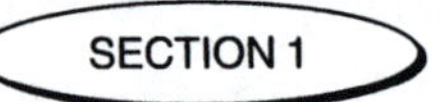

American Heart Association Treatment Algorithms

Adult Emergency Cardiac Care

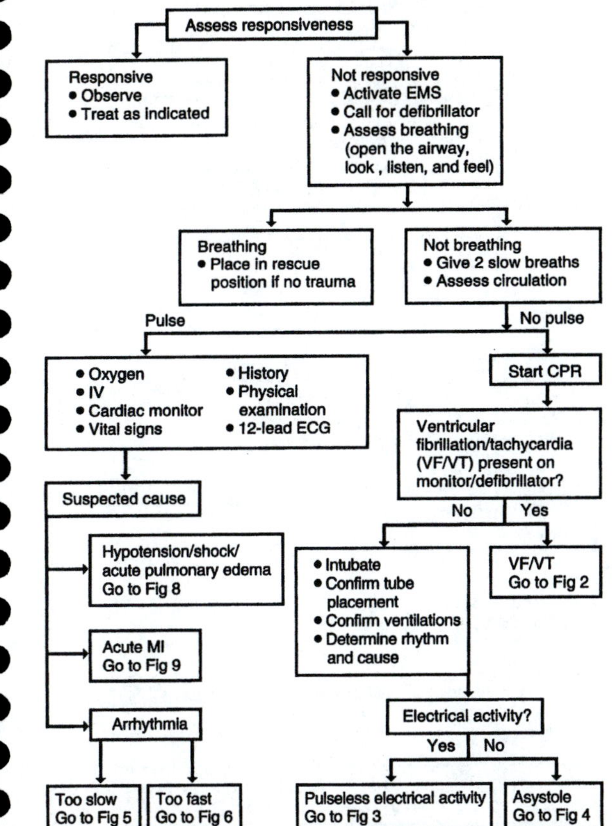

Figure 1. Universal algorithm for adult emergency cardiac care (ECC). (Reproduced with permission from Guidelines for Cardiopulmonary Resuscitation and Emergency Cardiac Care. Recommendations of the 1992 National Conference. American Heart Association. JAMA 268(16):2171–2302, October 28, 1992. Copyright 1992, American Medical Association.)

Ventricular Fibrillation and Pulseless Ventricular Tachycardia

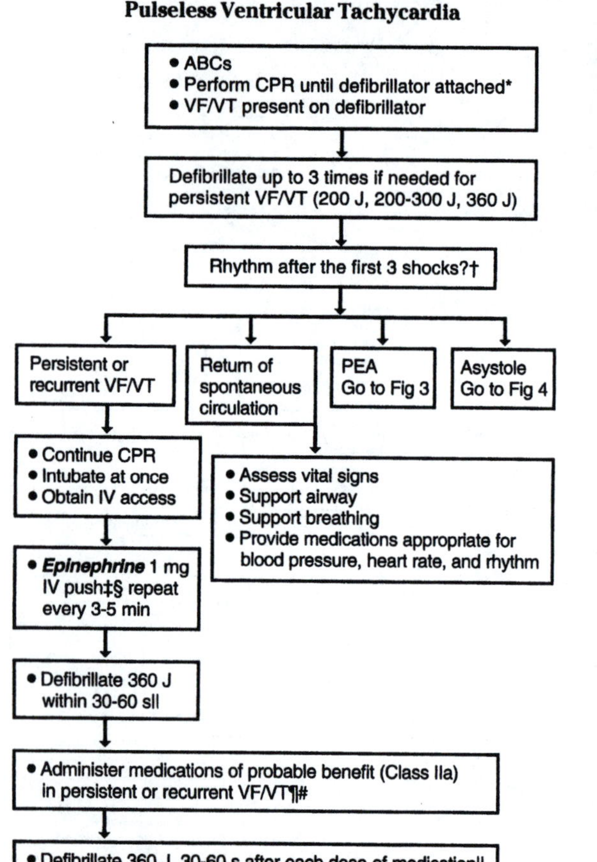

Figure 2. Algorithm for ventricular fibrillation and pulseless ventricular tachycardia (VF/VT). (Reproduced with permission from Guidelines for Cardiopulmonary Resuscitation and Emergency Cardiac Care. Recommendations of the 1992 National Conference. American Heart Association. JAMA 268(16):2171–2302, October 28, 1992. Copyright 1992, American Medical Association.)

Class I: definitely helpful
Class IIa: acceptable, probably helpful
Class IIb: acceptable, possibly helpful
Class III: not indicated, may be harmful
*Precordial thump is a Class IIb action in witnessed arrest, no pulse, and no defibrillator immediately available.
†Hypothermic cardiac arrest is treated differently after this point. See section on hypothermia.
‡The recommended dose of **epinephrine** is 1 mg IV push every 3-5 min. If this approach fails, several Class IIb dosing regimens can be considered:
- Intermediate: **epinephrine** 2-5 mg IV push, every 3-5 min
- Escalating: **epinephrine** 1 mg-3 mg-5 mg IV push (3 min apart)
- High: **epinephrine** 0.1 mg/kg IV push, every 3-5 min
§ **Sodium bicarbonate** (1 mEq/kg) is Class I if patient has known preexisting hyperkalemia
‖Multiple sequenced shocks (200J, 200-300J, 360 J) are acceptable here (Class I), especially when medications are delayed

¶ • **Lidocaine** 1.5 mg/kg IV push. Repeat in 3-5 min to total loading dose of 3 mg/kg; then use
- **Bretylium** 5 mg/kg IV push. Repeat in 5 min at 10 mg/kg
- **Magnesium sulfate** 1-2 g IV in torsades de pointes or suspected hypomagnesemic state or severe refractory VF
- **Procainamide** 30 mg/min in refractory VF (maximum total 17 mg/kg)

• **Sodium bicarbonate** (1 mEq/kg IV):
Class IIa
- if known preexisting bicarbonate-responsive acidosis
- if overdose with tricyclic antidepressants
- to alkalinize the urine in drug overdoses

Class IIb
- if intubated and continued long arrest interval
- upon return of spontaneous circulation after long arrest interval

Class III
- hypoxic lactic acidosis

Figure 2. (*continued*)

Pulseless Electrical Activity

PEA includes
- Electromechanical dissociation (EMD)
- Pseudo-EMD
- Idioventricular rhythms
- Ventricular escape rhythms
- Bradyasystolic rhythms
- Postdefibrillation idioventricular rhythms

- Continue CPR
- Intubate at once
- Obtain IV access
- Assess blood flow using Doppler ultrasound

↓

Consider possible causes
(Parentheses=possible therapies and treatments)
- Hypovolemia (volume infusion)
- Hypoxia (ventilation)
- Cardiac tamponade (pericardiocentesis)
- Tension pneumothorax (needle decompression)
- Hypothermia (see hypothermia algorithm, Section IV)
- Massive pulmonary embolism (surgery, *thrombolytics*)
- Drug overdoses such as tricyclics, digitalis, β-blockers, calcium channel blockers
- Hyperkalemia*
- Acidosis†
- Massive acute myocardial infarction (go to Fig 9)

↓

- *Epinephrine* 1 mg IV push, *‡ repeat every 3-5 min

↓

- If absolute bradycardia (<60 beats/min) or relative bradycardia, give *atropine* 1 mg IV
- Repeat every 3-5 min up to a total of 0.04 mg/kg§

Figure 3. Algorithm for pulseless electrical activity (PEA) (electromechanical dissociation [EMD]). (Reproduced with permission from Guidelines for Cardiopulmonary Resuscitation and Emergency Cardiac Care Recommendations of the 1992 National Conference. American Heart Sssociation. JAMA 268(16):2171–2302, October 28, 1992. Copyright 1992, American Medical Association.)

Class I: definitely helpful
Class IIa: acceptable, probably helpful
Class IIb: acceptable, possibly helpful
Class III: not indicated, may be harmful
*__Sodium bicarbonate__ 1 mEq/kg is Class I if patient has known preexisting
  hyperkalemia.
†__Sodium bicarbonate__ 1 mEq/kg:
  Class IIa
  • if known preexisting bicarbonate-responsive acidosis
  • if overdose with tricyclic antidepressants
  • to alkalinize the urine in drug overdoses
    Class IIb
  • if intubated and long arrest interval
  • upon return of spontaneous circulation after long arrest interval
    Class III
  • hypoxic lactic acidosis
‡The recommended dose of __epinephrine__ is 1 mg IV push every 3-5 min.
  If this approach fails, several Class IIb dosing regimens can be considered.
  • Intermediate: __epinephrine__ 2-5 mg IV push, every 3-5 min
  • Escalating: __epinephrine__ 1 mg-3 mg-5 mg IV push (3 min apart)
  • High: __epinephrine__ 0.1 mg/kg IV push, every 3-5 min
§ Shorter __atropine__ dosing intervals are possibly helpful
  in cardiac arrest (Class IIb).

Figure 3. (*continued*)

Asystole Treatment

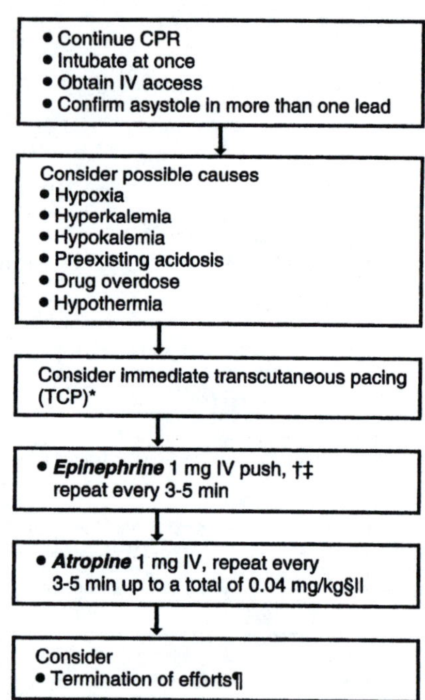

Figure 4. Asystole treatment algorithm. (Reproduced with permission from Guidelines for Cardiopulmonary Resuscitation and Emergency Cardiac Care. Recommendations of the 1992 National Conference. American Heart Association. JAMA 268(16):2171–2302, October 28, 1992. Copyright 1992, American Medical Association.)

Class I: definitely helpful
Class IIa: acceptable, probably helpful
Class IIb: acceptable, possibly helpful
Class III: not indicated, may be harmful

*TCP is a Class IIb intervention. Lack of success may be due to delays in pacing. To be effective TCP must be performed early, simultaneously with drugs. Evidence does not support routine use of TCP for asystole.

†The recommended dose of **epinephrine** is 1 mg IV push every 3-5 min. If this approach fails, several Class IIb dosing regimens can be considered:
- Intermediate: **epinephrine** 2-5 mg IV push, every 3-5 min
- Escalating: **epinephrine** 1 mg-3 mg-5 mg IV push (3 min apart)
- High: **epinephrine** 0.1 mg/kg IV push, every 3-5 min

‡**Sodium bicarbonate** 1 mEq/kg is Class I if patient has known preexisting hyperkalemia.

§Shorter **atropine** dosing intervals are Class IIb in asystolic arrest.

‖**Sodium bicarbonate** 1 mEq/kg:
Class IIa
- if known preexisting bicarbonate-responsive acidosis
- if overdose with tricyclic antidepressants
- to alkalinize the urine in drug overdoses

Class IIb
- if intubated and continued long arrest interval
- upon return of spontaneous circulation after long arrest interval

Class III
- hypoxic lactic acidosis

¶If patient remains in asystole or other agonal rhythms after successful intubation and initial medications and no reversible causes are identified, consider termination of resuscitative efforts by a physician. Consider interval since arrest.

Figure 4. (*continued*)

Bradycardia (Patient not in Cardiac Arrest)

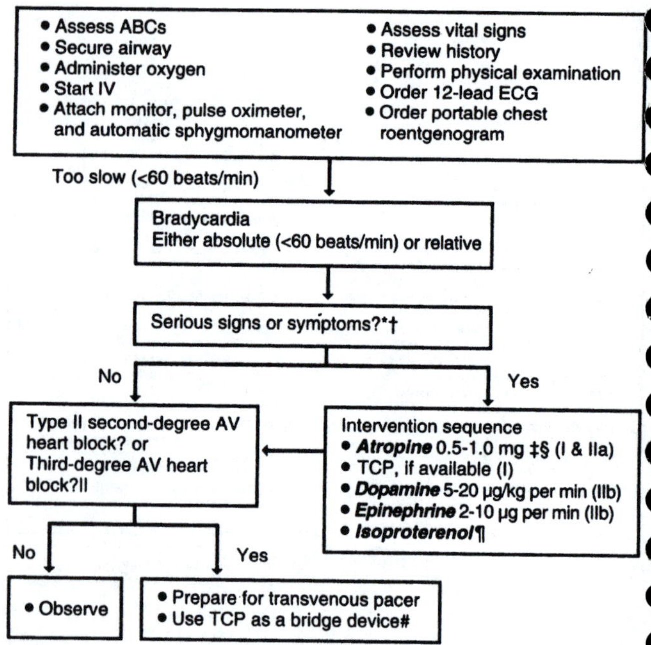

Figure 5. Bradycardia algorithm (with the patient not in cardiac arrest). (Reproduced with permission from Guidelines for Cardiopulmonary Resuscitation and Emergency Cardiac Care. Recommendations of the 1992 National Conference. American Heart Association. JAMA 268(16):2171–2302, October 28, 1992. Copyright 1992, American Medical Association.)

*Serious signs or symptoms must be related to the slow rate.
  Clinical manifestations include:
  symptoms (chest pain, shortness of breath, decreased level of
  conciousness) and
  signs (low BP, shock, pulmonary congestion, CHF, acute MI).
†Do not delay TCP while awating IV access or for ***atropine*** to take
  effect if patient is symptomatic.
‡Denervated transplanted hearts will not respond to ***atropine***. Go at once
  to pacing, ***catecholamine*** infusion, or both.
§***Atropine*** should be given in repeat doses in 3-5 min up to total of 0.04
  mg/kg. Consider shorter dosing intervals in severe clinical conditions.
  It has been suggested that atropine should be used with caution in
  atrioventricular (AV) block at the His-Purkinje level (type II AV block
  and new third-degree block with wide QRS complexes) (Class IIb).
‖Never treat third-degree heart block plus ventricular escape
  beats with ***lidocaine***.
¶***Isoproterenol*** should be used, if at all, with exteme caution. At low doses
  it is Class IIb (possibly helpful); at higher doses it is Class III (harmful).
#Verify patient tolerance and mechanical capture. Use analgesia and
  sedation as needed.

Figure 5. (*continued*)

Tachycardia

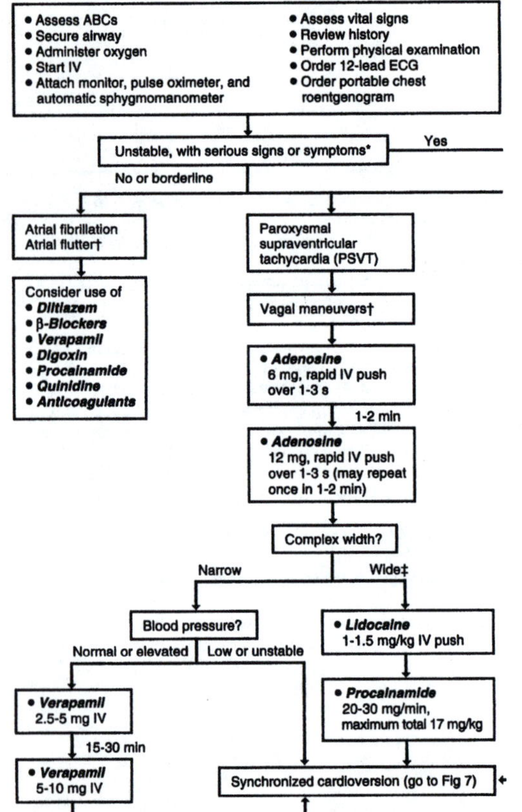

Figure 6. Tachycardia algorithm. (Reproduced with permission from Guidelines for Cardiopulmonary Resuscitation and Emergency Cardiac Care. Recommendations of the 1992 National Conference. American Heart Association. JAMA 268(16):2171–2302, October 28, 1992. Copyright 1992, American Medical Association.)

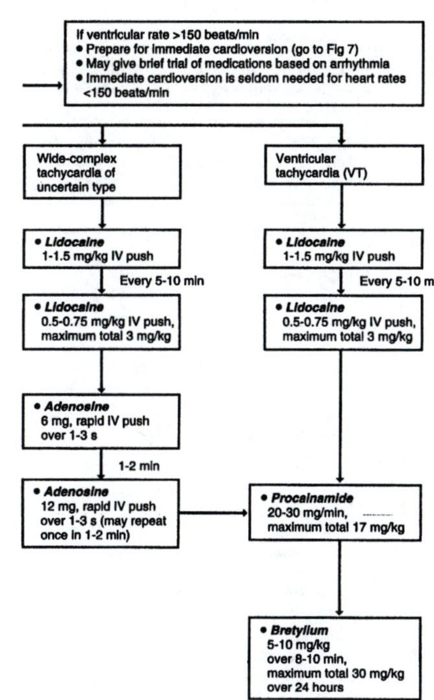

1

*Unstable condition must be related to the tachycardia. Signs and symptoms may include chest pain, shortness of breath, decreased level of consciousness, low blood pressure (BP), shock, pulmonary congestion, congestive heart failure, acute myocardial infarction.
†Carotid sinus pressure is contraindicated in patients with carotid bruits; avoid ice water immersion in patients with ischemic heart disease.
‡If the wide-complex tachycardia is known with certainty to be PSVT and BP is normal/elevated, sequence can include *verapamil.*

Figure 6. (*continued*)

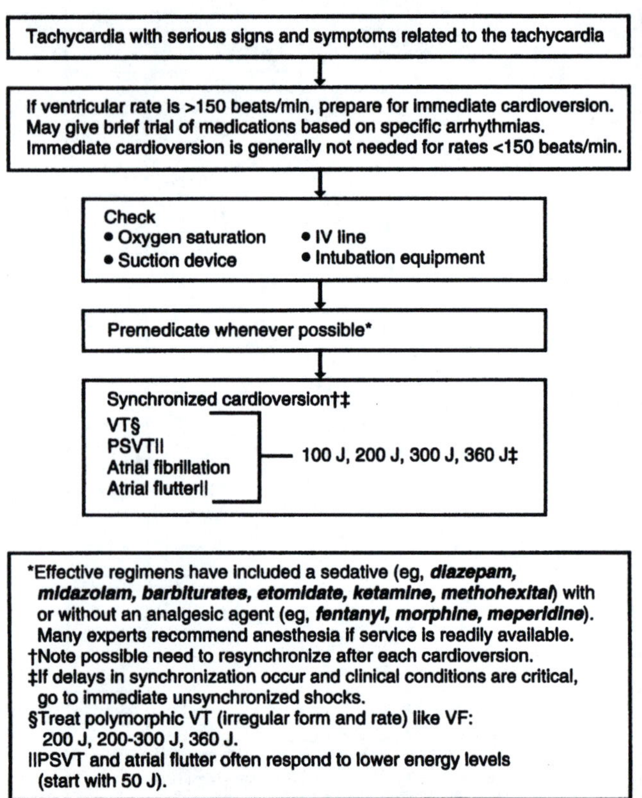

*Effective regimens have included a sedative (eg, *diazepam, midazolam, barbiturates, etomidate, ketamine, methohexital*) with or without an analgesic agent (eg, *fentanyl, morphine, meperidine*). Many experts recommend anesthesia if service is readily available.
†Note possible need to resynchronize after each cardioversion.
‡If delays in synchronization occur and clinical conditions are critical, go to immediate unsynchronized shocks.
§Treat polymorphic VT (irregular form and rate) like VF: 200 J, 200-300 J, 360 J.
‖PSVT and atrial flutter often respond to lower energy levels (start with 50 J).

Figure 7. Electrical cardioversion algorithm (with the patient not in cardiac arrest). (Reproduced with permission from Guidelines for Cardiopulmonary Resuscitation and Emergency Cardiac Care. Recommendations of the 1992 National Conference. American Heart Association. JAMA 268(16):2171–2302, October 28, 1992. Copyright 1992, American Medical Association.)

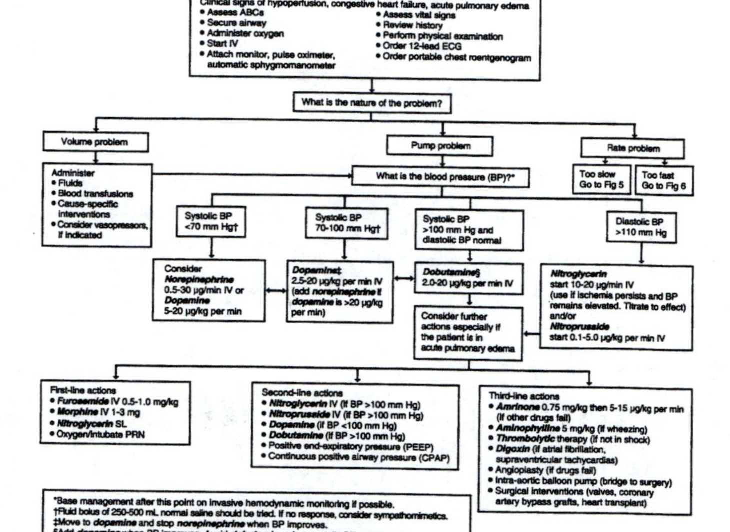

Figure 8. Algorithm for hypotension, shock, and acute pulmonary edema. (Reproduced with permission from Guidelines for Cardiopulmonary Resuscitation and Emergency Cardiac Care. Recommendations of the 1992 National Conference. American Heart Association. JAMA 268(16):2171–2302, October 28, 1992. Copyright 1992, American Medical Association.)

Acute Myocardial Infarction

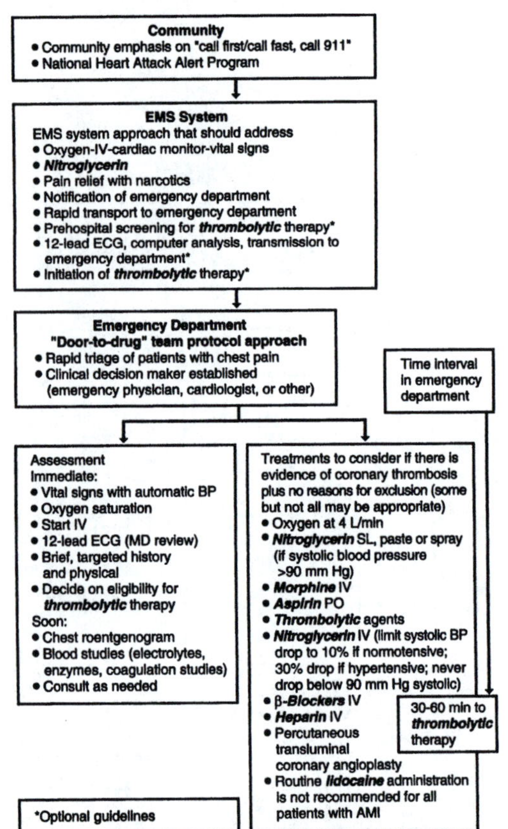

Figure 9. Acute myocardial infarction (AMI) algorithm. Recommendations for early treatment of patients with chest pain and possible AMI. (Reproduced with permission from Guidelines for Cardiopulmonary Resuscitation and Emergency Cardiac Care. Recommendations of the 1992 National Conference. American Heart Association. JAMA 268(16):2171–2302, October 28, 1992. Copyright 1992, American Medical Association.)

Pharmacology

2

Activated Charcoal (Arm-a-char, InstaChar)

Action: adsorbs ingested poisons, inhibiting their absorption in the GI tract.

Use: treatment of poisoning and overdoses in the alert patient after stomach has been emptied.

Contraindications: cyanide, mineral acids, strong bases, methanol, ethanol.

Route/Dosage: 30–60 g (5–10 tbs) mixed in water, PO.

Adverse Reactions/Side Effects: diarrhea, vomiting.

Adenosine (Adenocard)

Action: slows conduction through AV node of the heart.

Use: conversion of PSVT to NSR.

Contraindications: sick sinus syndrome, second- or third-degree heart block.

Route/Dosage: 6 mg rapid IVP. May repeat at 12 mg rapid IVP if necessary. May repeat 12 mg rapid IVP a third time if necessary.

Adverse Reactions/Side Effects: bronchoconstriction, dyspnea, palpitations, hypotension, chest pain, facial flushing, headache.

Albuterol (Proventil, Ventolin)

Action: bronchodilator (beta$_2$-adrenergic agonist).

Use: treatment of reversible airway obstruction.

Use Cautiously in: heart disease, hypertension, diabetes, elderly patients.

Route/Dosage: 2 inhalations q 4–6 h (90 µg/spray).

Adverse Reactions/Side Effects: hypertension, arrhythmias, chest pain, headache, nervousness.

Alteplase, Tissue Plasminogen Activator—t-PA (Activase)

Action: thrombolytic; dissolves thrombi, limiting infarction size during a myocardial infarction (MI).

Use: treatment of acute myocardial infarction (AMI) within 6 h of the onset of chest pain.

Contraindications: major surgery within 6 weeks, GI bleeding within 6 months, intracranial neoplasm, active bleeding, head trauma within 1 month, pregnancy.

Route/Dosage: 100 mg IV over 3 h as follows:
- 15 mg over 2 min
- 50 mg over 30 min (0.75 mg/kg)
- 35 mg over 60 min (0.5 mg/kg)

Adverse Reactions/Side Effects: reperfusion arrhythmias, intracranial bleeding, headache, hypotension, GI bleeding.

Aminophylline (Aminophyllin, Somophyllin)

Action: bronchodilator, relaxes bronchial smooth muscle, stimulates the heart.

Use: treatment of asthma, COPD, pulmonary edema, CHF.

Contraindications: uncontrolled cardiac arrhythmias.

Route/Dosage: 250–500 mg (5–6 mg/kg) added to 50–100 mL of D_5W and given IV over 20–30 min. Note: Rapid infusion (> 25 mg/min) can cause ventricular fibrillation.

Adverse Reactions/Side Effects: anxiety, headache, seizures, arrhythmias, tachycardia, palpitations.

Amrinone (Inocor)

Action: positive inotropic, vasodilator; decreases both preload and afterload.

Use: treatment of severe CHF that has not responded to milder agents.

Contraindications: hypersensitivity to bisulfite drugs. Note: Amrinone is incompatible with dextrose and furosemide. However, it may be given into a free-flowing IV line that contains a dextrose solution.

Route/Dosage: 0.75 mg/kg IVP over 2–3 min followed by an IV infusion of 5–15 µg/kg/min titrated to effect. Add 100 mg to 500 mL of NS, which yields a concentration of 0.2 mg/mL.

Adverse Reactions/Side Effects: arrhythmias, hypotension.

Amyl Nitrite

Action: cyanide poisoning adjunct; degrades cyanide by converting hemoglobin into methemoglobin.

Use: treatment of cyanide poisoning. Amyl nitrite is the first step in a three-step treatment for cyanide poisoning. After amyl nitrite, give sodium nitrite, then sodium thiosulfate.

Contraindications: none.

Route/Dosage: 1–2 ampules crushed and contents inhaled for 30 sec. Repeat until arrival at emergency department.

Adverse Reactions/Side Effects: severe headache, dizziness, weakness, muscle twitching, orthostatic hypotension, tachycardia, fainting, cold sweats.

Atropine

Action: antiarrhythmic, anticholinergic-antimuscarinic, organophosphate poisoning antidote; blocks action of acetylcholine in the parasympathetic nervous system.

Use: treatment of the following:

- Symptomatic sinus bradycardia
- AV block at the nodal level
- Ventricular asystole
- Slow PEA (absolute bradycardia [<60 beats/min] or relative brady-cardia)
- Organophosphate poisoning (antidote)

Contraindications: acute hemorrhage.

Route/Dosage:

- Symptomatic sinus bradycardia/AV block at the nodal level: 0.5–1.0 mg IVP. May repeat q 3–5 min to a total dose of 0.04 mg/kg.
- Asystole: 1 mg IVP. May repeat q 3–5 min to a total dose of 0.04 mg/kg.
- Atropine can be given via the ETT at 2–2.5 times the IVP dose.
- Organophosphate poisoning: 1 mg initially. If no improvement, give 2–5 mg IVP. Medical control may order additional doses while en route. In addition, pralidoxime may be necessary.

Adverse Reactions/Side Effects: drowsiness, confusion, tachycardia, VT, VF, blurred vision, dilated pupils, dry eyes, dry mouth.

Bretylium Tosylate (Bretylol)

Action: ventricular antiarrhythmic; initially causes a release of norepinephrine, followed in approximately 20 min by adrenergic blockage of norepinephrine.

Use: treatment of VT, VF, or wide-complex tachycardias of unknown origin in the following situations:

- When defibrillation, epinephrine, and lidocaine have failed to convert VF
- When lidocaine and procainamide have failed to control VT with a pulse
- When lidocaine, adenosine, and procainamide have failed to control wide-complex tachycardias of uncertain type

Contraindications: none.

Route/Dosage:
- VF/Pulseless VT: 5 mg/kg IVP. Can be repeated at 10 mg/kg IVP to a maximum dosage of 35 mg/kg.
- VT/Wide-complex tachycardias: 5–10 mg/kg IV infusion over 8–10 min.

Adverse Reactions/Side Effects: dizziness, syncope, vertigo, hypotension (may be significant, requiring infusion of IV replacement fluids), bradycardia angina, temporary hypertension.

Bumetanide (Bumex)

Action: inhibits the reabsorption of sodium and chloride in the kidneys; causes diuresis and works to lower blood pressure.

Use: treatment of the following:
- Edema secondary to CHF
- Hypertension

Contraindications: known hypersensitivity to bumetanide.

Precautions: Use with caution in patients whose electrolytes are depleted or patients who have diabetes mellitus.

Route/Dosage: 0.5–2 mg IM or over 2 min by IV bolus.

Adverse Reactions/Side Effects: headache, dizziness, hypotension, possible ECG changes, metabolic alkalosis, hypovolemia, dehydration.

Butorphanol (Stadol)

Action: alters the awareness of and response to pain.

Use: treatment of moderate to severe pain.

Contraindications: do not use in patients who:
- Are dependent on opiates
- Have suffered head injury
- Complain of abdominal pain

Route/Dosage:
- IV bolus: 0.5–2 mg q 3 h as needed
- IM: 1–4 mg q 3 h as needed

Adverse Reactions/Side Effects: headache, hallucinations, hypotension/hypertension, palpitations, respiratory depression.
Contraindications: during resuscitative efforts unless hyperkalemia, hypocalcemia, or calcium channel blocker toxicity has been documented.
Route/Dosage:
- Calcium chloride: 2–4 mg/kg slow IVP; may be repeated q 10 min if needed
- Calcium gluceptate: 5–7 mL slow IVP
- Calcium gluconate: 5–8 mL slow IVP

Adverse Reactions/Side Effects: syncope, cardiac arrest, arrhythmias, bradycardia.

Calcium Salts; Calcium Chloride (10%), Calcium Gluceptate, Calcium Gluconate

Action: electrolyte modifier; essential for the transmission of nerve impulses that initiate the contraction of cardiac muscle.
Use: balance of severe excesses of potassium (hyperkalemia) or severe deficits of calcium (hypocalcemia) in the blood.
Contraindications: not to be used during resuscitation unless hyperkalemia, hypocalcemia, or calcium channel blocker toxicity has been proven.
Route/Dosage:
- Calcium chloride: 2–4 mg/kg slow IVP, may be repeated q 5 min as needed
- Calcium gluceptate: 5–7 mL slow IVP
- Calcium gluconate: 5–8 mL slow IVP

Adverse Reactions/ Side Effects: syncope, arrhythmias, bradycardia, cardiac arrest, tissue necrosis at injection site.

Dexamethasone (Decadron, Hexadrol)

Action: anti-inflammatory; suppresses inflammation.
Use: treatment of shock, acute cerebral edema, and severe allergic reactions.
Contraindications: none.
Route/Dosage:
- Shock: 100 mg (1–6 mg/kg) slow IVP
- Cerebral edema: 10 mg slow IVP
- Severe allergic reactions: 4 mg slow IVP

Adverse Reactions/Side Effects: headache, depression,

restlessness, hypertension, increased intracranial pressure, fluid retention, hypokalemia.

Dextrose 50% in Water/$D_{50}W$

Action: hyperglycemic; increases circulating blood sugar levels. Some EMS protocols recommend $D_{50}W$ in certain cardiac arrest situations.
Use: treatment of the following:
- Coma caused by hypoglycemia
- Coma of unknown cause
- Altered LOC with reagent strip reading <45 mg

Contraindications: intracranial hemorrhage.
Route/Dosage: 25 g slow IVP. Repeat if needed.
Adverse Reactions/Side Effects: may cause CNS symptoms in the alcoholic patient; may aggravate hypertension and CHF; may cause tissue necrosis at the injection site.

Diazepam (Valium, Valrelease)

Action: antianxiety agent, anticonvulsant, skeletal muscle relaxant; causes CNS depression.
Use: treatment of the following:
- Status epilepticus and major motor seizures
- Seizures caused by cocaine overdose

Also used as a skeletal muscle relaxant and for sedation before cardioversion.
Route/Dosage:
- Seizures/muscle relaxant: 2–5 mg slow IVP. Repeat as needed, but do not exceed a total dose of 10 mg.
- Status epilepticus: 5–10 mg slow IVP. Repeat q 10–15 min if needed, to a maximum dose of 30 mg.
- Seizures caused by cocaine overdose: CNS overstimulation—2.5–5 mg slow IVP; active seizures 5–10 mg slow IVP.
- Sedation before cardioversion: 5–15 mg slow IVP.

Adverse Reactions/Side Effects: drowsiness, mental depression, headache, hypotension, respiratory depression, blurred vision, increased intraocular pressure.

Diazoxide (Hyperstat, Proglycem)

Action: antihypertensive; causes vasodilation and decreases peripheral vascular resistance.

Use: treatment of malignant hypertension.
Contraindications: known hypersensitivity to thiazide diuretics.
Route/Dosage: 1–3 mg/kg, up to 150 mg single rapid IVP. Repeat in
  5–15 min if needed.
Adverse Reactions/Side Effects: headache, light-headedness,
  tachycardia, hypotension, arrhythmia, chest pain, edema, CHF,
  sodium and water retention.

Digoxin (Lanoxin)

Action: antiarrhythmic, inotropic; increases both force and velocity of
  ventricular contractions while slowing conduction through the AV
  node.
Use: treatment of the following:
- Atrial fibrillation
- Atrial flutter
- PSVT
- CHF

Many EMS protocols do not permit out-of-hospital use of digoxin.
Contraindications: uncontrolled ventricular arrhythmias
Route/Dosage: 10–15 µg/kg slow IVP. Should be given in divided
  doses to avoid toxicity. Consult protocols.
Adverse Reactions/Side Effects: fatigue, headache, blurred vision,
  yellow vision, bradycardia, almost any cardiac arrhythmia.

Diphenhydramine (Benadryl, Benylin)

Action: antihistamine (H_1 receptor antagonist); blocks the effects of
  histamine.
Use: in addition to epinephrine, treatment of allergic symptoms caused
  by histamine release.
Contraindications: acute asthma attacks.
Route/Dosage: 10–50 mg slow IVP or deep IM.
Adverse Reactions/Side Effects: drowsiness, dizziness, headache,
  (possibly) paradoxic excitement in children, wheezing, thickening
  of bronchial secretions, tightness of chest, palpitations, hypotension,
  blurred vision.

Dobutamine (Dobutrex)

Action: inotropic agent increasing cardiac contractility and stroke
  volume.

Use: treatment of the following:
- Pulmonary congestion and low cardiac output
- Hypotensive patients with pulmonary congestion who cannot tolerate vasodilators

Contraindications: tachyarrhythmias.

Route/Dosage: 2–20 µg/kg/min IV infusion titrated to effect. Prepare infusion → add 250 mg to 250 mL of D_5W or NS (1000 µg/mL).

Adverse Reactions/Side Effects: headache, tachycardia, hypertension, PVCs, chest pain, shortness of breath.

Dopamine (Dopastat, Intropin)

Action: inotropic, vasopressor; increases blood pressure and cardiac output, and improves blood flow through the kidneys.

Use: treatment of hemodynamically significant hypotension in the absence of hypovolemia.

Contraindications: pheochromocytoma.

Route/Dosage: 2.5–5 µg/kg/min IV infusion. Increase infusion rate until therapeutic effect is seen.
- Vasodilation of renal, mesenteric, and cerebral arteries: 1–2 µg/kg/min
- Increased cardiac output (beta): 2–10 µg/kg/min
- Vasoconstriction (alpha): 10–20 µg/kg/min
- Vasoconstriction, positive inotropism: >20 µg/kg/min

Prepare infusion by adding: 400 mg 250 mL of D5W or 800 mg 500 mL of D_5W, producing a concentration of 1600 µg/mL.

Adverse Reactions/Side Effects: arrhythmias, hypotension, palpitations, chest pain, dyspnea, dilated pupils, tissue necrosis at IV site.

Epinephrine 1:1000/1:10,000 (Adrenalin)

Action: bronchodilator, cardiac stimulator, peripheral vasoconstrictor; stimulates both alpha- and beta-adrenergic receptors.

Use: treatment of the following:
- Cardiac arrest (VF, pulseless, VT, asystole, PEA)
- Symptomatic sinus bradycardia
- Bronchial asthma
- Anaphylaxis

Contraindications: none during cardiac arrest; otherwise, shock, arrhythmias.

Route/Dosage:
- Cardiac arrest: 1 mg IVP q 3–5 min during the arrest. Dosage options include the following:
  - ○ Intermediate: 2–5 mg IVP q 3–5 min
  - ○ Escalating: 1 mg–3 mg–5 mg IVP 3 min apart
  - ○ High: 0.1 mg/kg IVP q 3–5 min

Note: Epinephrine can be given via the ETT at 2–2.5 times the IVP dosage.
- Symptomatic sinus bradycardia: 1 µg/min IV infusion titrated to effect. Prepare infusion by adding 1 mg (1 mL) of a 1:1000 sol to 500 mL of NS of D_5W (2 µg/mL).
- Bronchial asthma: 0.3–0.5 mg (0.3–0.5 mL) SC (1:1000 sol)
- Anaphylaxis (mild/moderate): 0.3–0.5 mg SC (1:1000 sol)
- Anaphylaxis (severe): 0.3–0.5 mg (3–5 mL) IVP (1:10,000 sol). May require an infusion at 1–4 µg/min. Prepare infusion by adding 2 mg (1:1000 sol) to 500 mL of D_5W (4 µg/mL).

Adverse Reactions/Side Effects: nervousness, restlessness, headache, tremors, arrhythmias, angina, hypertension.

Ethacrynic Acid (Edecrin)

Action: diuretic; reduces edema and lowers blood pressure.
Use: treatment of the following:
- Edema secondary to CHF
- Hypertension

Contraindications: do not give to patients who are hypotensive.
Route/Dosage: 0.5–1 mg/kg or 50–100 mg IV bolus. A single dose should not exceed 100 mg.
Adverse Reactions/Side Effects: headache, dizziness, hypotension, hypovolemia, metabolic alkalosis, dehydration.

Furosemide (Lasix)

Action: antihypertensive, diuretic; inhibits the reabsorption of sodium and chloride in the kidneys.
Use: treatment of lung congestion associated with inadequate ventricular function.
Contraindications: hypotension, hypokalemia.
Route/Dosage: 0.5–1.0 mg/kg slow IVP.
Adverse Reactions/Side Effects: dizziness, headache, hypotension, arrhythmias, potassium depletion, metabolic alkalosis.

Glucagon

Action: antihypoglycemic; increases the level of circulating blood
   sugar.
Use: treatment of hypoglycemia in an unconscious patient, a
   combative patient, or a patient in whom an IV cannot be started.
Contraindications: none.
Route/Dosage: 0.5–1.0 U 1M, SC, or IV.
Adverse Reactions/Side Effects: dizziness, possible hypotension.

Haloperidol (Haldol)

Action: antipsychotic; blocks the effects of dopamine in the CNS.
Use: treatment of acute and chronic psychoses.
Contraindications: CNS depression, circulatory compromise.
Route/Dosage: 2–5 mg IM.
Adverse Reactions/Side Effects: sedation, confusion, restlessness,
   seizures, respiratory depression.

Hydralazine (Apresoline)

Action: antihypertensive; causes dilation of peripheral arterioles.
Use: treatment of moderate to severe hypertension and CHF resistant to
   digitalis glycosides and diuretics.
Contraindications: coronary artery disease, mitral-valve rheumatic
   heart disease.
Route/Dosage: 20–40 mg slow IVP or IM.
Adverse Reactions/Side Effects: dizziness, drowsiness,
   tachycardia, arrhythmias, orthostatic hypotension, chest pain.

Hydrocortisone (Cortef, Cortisol, Hydrocortone, Solu-Cortef)

Action: anti-inflammatory; replaces cortisol in deficiency states.
Use: short-term management of allergic reactions.
Contraindications: none.
Route/Dosage: 100–500 mg IVP. Dilute 100 mg in 50–100 mL of D_5W or
   NS.
Adverse Reactions/Side Effects: depression, euphoria, increased
   intraocular pressure, sodium retention, hypokalemia.

Hydromorphone (Dilaudid)

Action: analgesic, antitussive; alters the awareness of and response to
   pain, causes CNS depression, suppresses cough.

Use: treatment of moderate to severe pain.

Contraindications: head traumia, abdominal pain, pulmonary disease.

Route/Dosage: 1 mg slow IVP. Repeat 0.5–1.0 mg q 5 min until adequate pain relief or respiratory depression occurs.

Adverse Reactions/Side Effects: headache, confusion, dizziness, sedation, hypotension, bradycardia, respiratory depression.

Hydroxyzine (Atarax, Vistaril)

Action: antianxiety agent, sedative; causes sedation and relief of anxiety.

Use: treatment of anxiety.

Contraindications: none.

Route/Dosage: 50–100 mg deep IM.

Adverse Reactions/Side Effects: drowsiness, dizziness, weakness, headache, wheezing, chest tightness.

Insulin—Animal-Derived or Biosynthetic (Humulin, Iletin, Novolin)

Action: helps to control blood sugar levels in patients with diabetes.

Use: treatment of diabetic ketoacidosis (severe hyperglycemia).

Contraindications: hypersensitivity to beef or pork. In these cases, a biosynthetic insulin should be used.

Route/Dosage:

- Adult IV: 2–10 U (0.1 U/kg) loading dose, followed by 2–10 U (0.1 U/kg/h) by IV infusion. Add 100 U of regular insulin to 1000 mL of NS, giving a concentration of 0.1 U/mL.
- Adult IV SC: 25–150 U IV bolus initially. Give additional doses based on blood glucose levels OR 50–100 U by IV bolus plus 50–100 USC initially. Give additional SC doses q 2–6h as needed.

Adverse Reactions/Side Effects: itching, swelling, redness, hypoglycemia, allergic reactions.

Isoetharine (Arm-a-Med, Beta-2, Bisorine, Bronkosol, Dey-Dose, Dey-Lute, Dispose-a-Med)

Action: bronchodilator; relaxes smooth bronchial muscles.

Use: relief of dyspnea caused by asthma or COPD.

Contraindications: hypersensitivity to amine drugs.

Route/Dosage:
Inhalation: 1–2 inhalations (340 µg/spray)
- Oxygen aerosol: 0.25–0.5 mL of a 1% sol diluted 1:3. Other concentrations include the following:
  - o 2–4 mL of 0.125%
  - o 2.5 mL of 0.2%
  - o 2 mL of 0.25%
- Nebulization: four inhalations of a 0.5%–1% sol.

Adverse Reactions/Side Effects: nervousness, tremor, headache, dizziness, hypertension, arrhythmias, chest pain.

Isoproterenol (Isuprel)

Action: antiarrhythmic, bronchodilator, cardiac stimulator; causes increased cardiac output, improves blood return to the heart, and causes bronchodilation.

Use:
- Treatment of refractory torsade de pointes
- Immediate temporary control of hemodynamically significant bradycardia of heart transplant patients

Contraindications: ischemic heart disease, hypotension, cardiac arrest.

Route/Dosage: 2–10 µg/min IV infusion, titrated to effect. Add 1 mg to 500 mL of D_5W, producing a concentration of 2 µg/mL.

Adverse Reactions/Side Effects: nervousness, tremors, headache, serious arrhythmias, hypertension, angina.

Labetalol (Normodyne, Trandate)

Action: causes a decrease in heart rate and blood pressure.

Use: treatment of hypertension.

Contraindications: CHF, pulmonary edema, cardiogenic shock, bradycardia, heart block, pregnancy.

Route/Dosage:
- IV bolus: 20 mg over 2 min. Subsequent doses of 40–80 mg at 10 min intervals if needed. Total dose should not exceed 300 mg.
- IV infusion: 2 mg/min. Add 200 mg to 250 mL of D_5W, producing a concentration of 0.9 mg/ml. Run at 150 gtts/min.

Adverse Reactions/Side Effects: fatigue, depression, bradycardia, CHF, pulmonary edema, hypotension, bronchospasm, wheezing, blurred vision, dry eyes.

Lidocaine (Xylocaine)

Action: ventricular antiarrhythmic; decreases excessive spontaneous activity of ectopic pacemaker sites in the His-Purkinje fibers.

Use: treatment of the following:
- Ventricular ectopy in the presence of an AMI
- VT
- VF/pulseless VT

Contraindications: severe heart block. Adams-Stokes syndrome, Wolff-Parkinson-White syndrome.

Route/Dosage:
- VF/pulseless VT: 1.5 mg/kg IVP. Can be repeated in 3–5 min, to a total dose of 3 mg/kg. Upon spontaneous circulation, begin IV infusion at 2–4 mg/min. Add 2 g to 500 mL of D_5W, producing a concentration of 4 mg/mL (4:1 concentration). Infusion rates; 2 mg/min = 15 µgtts/min; 3 mg/min = 45 µgtts/min; 4 mg/min = 60 µgtts/min.
- VT: 1–1.5 mg/kg IVP. Can repeat at 0.5–0.75 mg/kg q 5–10 min to a total dose of 3 mg/kg. When VT has been corrected, begin IV infusion at 2–4 mg/min.
- PVCs in presence of AMI: 0.5 mg/kg IVP. May repeat to a total dose of 2 mg/kg.

Adverse Reactions/Side Effects: anxiety, drowsiness, confusion, seizures, respiratory arrest, hypotension, bradycardia, arrhythmias, cardiac arrest.

Lorazepam (Ativan)

Action: antianxiety agent; relieves anxiety and provides amnesia.

Use: sedation and relief of anxiety.

Contraindications: coma, pre-existing CNS depression, uncontrolled severe pain.

Route/Dosage:
- Mild agitation: 0.5–1.0 mg IV
- Moderate agitation: 1–2 mg IV
- Severe agitation: 2–4 mg IV

Adverse Reactions/Side Effects: dizziness, drowsiness, respiratory depression.

Magnesium Sulfate

Action:
- Cardiac: resolves magnesium-deficient states associated with sudden cardiac death.
- Pregnancy: resolves seizures associated with preeclampsia or eclampsia.

Use:
- Cardiac: treatment of the following:
  o Torsade de pointes
  o Refractory VF/pulseless VT
- Pregnancy: anticonvulsant in the prevention or control of seizures in preeclampsia or eclampsia.

Contraindications:
- Cardiac: hypocalcemia, heart block
- Pregnancy: heart block, respiratory depression

Route/Dosage:
- Cardiac: dilute 1–2 g in 100 mL of D_5W and give over 1–2 min
- Pregnancy: 2–4 g IV over 3 min. Follow with an IV infusion of 1–2 g/h

Adverse Reactions/Side Effects: drowsiness, respiratory depression, bradycardia, arrhythmias, hypotension.

Mannitol (Osmitrol)

Action: diuretic; inhibits the reabsorption of water and electrolytes.
Use: relief of excessive intracranial pressure.
Contraindications: pre-existing dehydration, active intracranial bleeding.
Route/Dosage: 1.5–2.0 g/kg of a 20% sol by IV infusion.
Adverse Reactions/Side Effects: headache, confusion, tachycardia, chest pain, CHF, pulmonary edema, blurred vision, dehydration.

Meperidine (Demerol)

Action: analgesic, alters awareness of and response to pain and causes generalized CNS depression.
Use: treatment of moderate to severe pain.
Contraindications: head injury, undiagnosed abdominal pain.

Route/Dosage:
- IV infusion: 15–35 mg/h. Add 50 mg to 500 mL of D_5W, producing a concentration of 0.1 mg/mL.
- IM: 50–100 mg q 3–4 h.

Adverse Reactions/Side Effects: headache, confusion, sedation, hallucinations, hypotension, bradycardia, respiratory depression.

Metaproterenol (Alupent, Metaprel)

Action: bronchodilator; relaxes smooth bronchial muscles, resulting in an increased lung capacity and a decrease in airway resistance.

Use: treatment of dyspnea caused by asthma or COPD.

Contraindications: pre-existing cardiac arrhythmias associated with tachycardia.

Route/Dosage:
- Inhalation: 2–3 inhalations q 3–4 h by metered-dose inhaler (650 µg/spray).
- Nebulization: 5–15 inhalations of an undiluted 5% sol 3–4 times/day. Also, 0.2–0.3 mL of a 5% sol diluted in 2.5 mL of NS, 3–4 times/day.

Adverse Reactions/Side Effects: headache, anxiety, fear, nervousness, palpitations, tachycardia, arrhythmias, respiratory weakness.

Methylprednisolone (A-methaPred, Medrol, Solu-Medrol)

Action:
- Neurologic: anti-inflammatory—protects nerve fibers and inhibits swelling, ischemia, nerve cell death, and electrolyte imbalance to the spinal cord caused by trauma.
- Anaphylaxis: suppresses inflammatory response and modifies the body's normal immune response.

Use:
- Neurologic: treatment of traumatic spinal cord injury with loss of motor function
- Anaphylaxis: treatment of severe anaphylaxis

Contraindications: none.

Route/Dosage:
- Neurologic: 30 mg/kg IVP, followed by IV infusion of 5.4 mg/kg/h
- Anaphylaxis: 100–200 mg IV or IM

Adverse Reactions/Side Effects: depression, euphoria, restlessness, headache, hypertension, increased intraocular pressure, hyperglycemia, hypokalemia, fluid retention.

Metoprolol (Lopressor)

Action: decreases heart rate and blood pressure.

Use:
- Treatment of hypertension
- Treatment of angina pectoris
- Early intervention in AMI

Contraindications: CHF, second- or third-degree heart block, bradycardia.

Route/Dosage: 5 mg slow IV bolus q 2 min for up to 3 doses or as long as vital signs remain stable.

Adverse Reactions/Side Effects: weakness, dizziness, depression, bradycardia, pulmonary edema, CHF, bronchospasm, wheezing, blurred vision.

Midazolam (Versed)

Action: sedative/hypnotic; provides conscious sedation/amnesia.

Use: short-term sedation.

Contraindications: shock, pre-existing CNS depression, uncontrolled severe pain.

Route/Dosage:
- Mild agitation: 1–2 mg IVP
- Moderate agitation: 5 mg IVP
- Severe agitation: 7–10 mg IVP

Adverse Reactions/Side Effects: headache, arrhythmias, cardiac arrest.

Morphine (Duramorph, Roxanol)

Action: narcotic analgesic; increases venous capacity and decreases systemic vascular resistance.

Use: treatment of the following:
- Pain and anxiety associated with AMI
- Acute cardiogenic pulmonary edema

Contraindications: hypotension, respiratory depression not associated with pulmonary edema, head injury, abdominal pain, patients on depressant drugs.

Route/Dosage: 1–3 mg slow IVP q 5–30 min until desired effect is achieved. Do not exceed 15 mg in the out-of-hospital setting.

Adverse Reactions/Side Effects: confusion, sedation, headache, hypotension, bradycardia, respiratory depression, dry eyes, blurred vision.

Nalbuphine (Nubain)

Action: alters the awareness of and response to pain.

Use: treatment of moderate to severe pain.

Contraindications: head trauma, increased intracranial pressure, undiagnosed abdominal pain.

Route/Dosage: 5–10 mg IV bolus initially. Repeat with 2 mg doses if needed.

Adverse Reactions/Side Effects: headache, dizziness, vertigo, confusion, hypotension, hypertension, palpitations, respiratory depression, dry mouth.

Naloxone (Narcan)

Action: narcotic antagonist; blocks narcotic analgesics, reversing their effects.

Use:

- Treatment of symptomatic narcotic overdose
- Diagnostic tool in coma of unknown origin

Contraindications: none.

Route/Dosage: 0.4–2.0 mg slow IVP, ET, SC, IM. Repeat q 2–3 min if needed.

Adverse Reactions/Side Effects: VT, VF, hypotension, hypertension. May cause withdrawal syndrome in the narcotic-dependent patient.

Nifedipine (Adalat, Procardia)

Action: antianginal; decreases afterload, thereby decreasing myocardial oxygen consumption.

Use: treatment of the following:

- Angina pectoris
- Hypertensive crisis

Contraindications: heart block.

Route/Dosage: 5–10 mg SL or 10–40 mg PO.

Adverse Reactions/Side Effects: headache, dizziness, nervousness, dyspnea, cough, wheezing, CHF, MI, ventricular arrhythmias, hypotension, syncope.

Nitroglycerin (Nitrostat, Nitro-bid, Nitro-Dur, Nitrolingual, Nitrol, NTG, Tridil)

Action: antianginal, coronary vasodilator; vasodilation causes decreased blood return to the heart.

Use: treatment of the following:
- Angina pectoris
- CHF

Contraindications: head trauma, hypotension, hypovolemia, shock.

Route/Dosage:
- SL: 0.3–0.4 mg tablet. Repeat q 5 min to a total dose of 0.9–1.2 mg.
- IVP: 50 µg, followed by IV infusion.
- IV infusion: 10–20 µg/min, increasing by 5–10 µg/min q 5–10 min to effect.
- Lingual spray: 0.4 mg/spray. Repeat q 3–5 min for a total of 3 sprays (1.2 mg).
- Ointment: 1–2 in (15–30 mg) q 8 h, up to 5 in q 4 h.
- Transdermal patch: 2.5–15 mg/24 h.

Adverse Reactions/Side Effects: headache, dizziness, weakness, hypotension, tachycardia, fainting.

Nitroprusside (Nipride, Nitropress)

Action: antihypertensive; increases the capacity of the venous circulation and reduces blood pressure.

Use: treatment of the following:
- Hypertensive crisis
- Acute heart failure
- Cardiogenic shock

Contraindications: decreased cerebral perfusion (some protocols state that there are no contraindications for a life-threatening hypertensive crisis).

Route/Dosage: 0.1–5.0 µg/kg/min IV infusion. Doses up to 10 µg/kg/min may be needed. Add 50 mg to 250–500 mL of D_5W producing a concentration of 200 µg/mL (250 mL) or 100 µg/mL (500 mL).

Adverse Reactions/Side Effects: headache, dizziness, palpitations, dyspnea, hypotension.

Nitrous Oxide–Oxygen Mixture (Entonox, Nitronox)

Action: analgesic; produces rapid but reversible relief from pain.

Use: patient-administered, relief of moderate to severe pain from any cause.

Contraindications: decreased level of consciousness, patients on depressant drugs, thoracic trauma, respiratory compromise, developing cyanosis, patient unable to follow simple instructions, abdominal distention or trauma, pregnancy.

Route/Dosage: self-administration by the patient until the pain is relieved.

Adverse Reactions/Side Effects: light-headedness, drowsiness, decreased respirations.

Norepinephrine (Levophed)

Action: vasopressor; increases both blood pressure and cardiac output.

Use: treatment of hemodynamically significant hypotension.

Contraindications: hypotension caused by hypovolemia, myocardial ischemia, or infarction.

Route/Dosage: 0.5–1.0 µg/min IV infusion initially. Can increase until a blood pressure of 90 mm Hg is achieved. Add 4 mg to 250 mL of D_5W or NS, producing a concentration of 16 µg/mL.

Adverse Reactions/Side Effects: headache, anxiety, dizziness, restlessness, bradycardia, hypertension, arrhythmias, chest pain, dyspnea.

Oxygen

Action: medicinal gas; increases arterial oxygen tension (Pao_2) and hemoglobin saturation.

Use: treatment of the following:

* Severe chest pain due to cardiac ischmia
* Hypoxemia from any cause
* Cardiac arrest

Contraindications: none.

Route/Dosage: inhalation. Some of the more common oxygen devices and their delivery capacities include the following:

* Nasal cannula: 1–6 L/min (24%–44%)
* Face mask: 8–10 L/min (40%–60%)
* Face mask with reservoir: 1–10 L/min (60%–almost 100%)

- Venturi mask:
  - 24% at 4 L/min
  - 28% at 4 L/min
  - 35% at 8 L/min
  - 40% at 8 L/min
- Mouth to mask: using supplemental oxygen at 10 L/min (50%).

Adverse Reactions/Side Effects: None. However, dry, nonhumidified oxygen can dry out mucous membranes, causing pain for the patient.

Oxytocin (Pitocin, Syntocinon)

Action: oxytocic; contracts uterine blood vessels.
Use: control of postartum hemorrhage.
Contraindications: none.
Route/Dosage:
- IV infusion: 10–20 U added to 1000 mL of LR or NS, titrated to control hemorrhage.
- IM: 3–10 U.

Adverse Reactions/Side Effects: seizures, coma, hypotension, arrhythmias, increased heart rate and cardiac output.

Pancuronium (Pavulon)

Action: neuromuscular blocking drug causing skeletal muscle paralysis.
Use: inducement of paralysis to facilitate intubation.
Contraindications: renal failure.
Route/Dosage: 0.04–0.1 mg/kg IV initially. Supplemental doses of 0.01 mg/kg may be given if needed.
Adverse Reactions/Side Effects: tachycardia, apnea, wheezing, excessive sweating (children), muscle weakness, excessive salivation (children).

Pentazocine (Talwin)

Action: analgesic; alters awareness of and response to pain.
Use: treatment of moderate to severe pain.
Contraindications: head injury, undiagnosed abdominal pain.
Route/Dosage:
- IVP: 30 mg initially. Can repeat q 3–4 h; do not exceed 360 mg.
- IM: 30–60 mg initially. Can repeat q 3–4 h; do not exceed 360 mg.

Adverse Reactions/Side Effects: headache, dizziness, sedation, hallucinations, euphoria, hypotension, hypertension, palpitations, respiratory depression.

Phenobarbital (Luminal)

Action: anticonvulsant, sedative, hypnotic; supresses the spread of seizure activity.

Use: treatment of seizures.

Contraindications: headache, vertigo, bronchospasm, laryngospasm respiratory depression, hypotension.

Route/Dosage:
- Anticonvulsant: 100–300 mg slow IVP
- Status epileptics: 10–20 mg/kg slow IVP

Adverse Reactions/Side Effects: drowsiness, headache, vertigo, bronchospasm, laryngospasm, respiratory depression, hypotension.

Pralidoxime (Protopam)

Action: antidote, anticholinesterase poisoning inhibitor; reverses paralysis caused by organophosphate poisoning.

Use: given after atropine in severe cases of organophosphate pesticide poisoning.

Contraindications: inorganic phosphates.

Route/Dosage: 1–2 g IV infusion over 30–60 min, after administering atropine. Add 1 g to 500 mL of NS, producing a concentration of 2 mg/mL.

Adverse Reactions/Side Effects: dizziness, headache, tachycardia, blurred vision.

Procainamide (Procan SR, Promine, Pronestyl, Pronestyl-SR)

Action: antiarrhythmic; slows conduction velocity in the bundle of His.

Use: treatment of the following:
- Refractory VF
- PSVT
- Wide-complex tachycardia of uncertain type
- VT

Contraindications: pre-existing QT prolongation, torsade de pointes.

Route/Dosage: 20–30 mg/min IV infusion until
- Arrhythmia has been suppressed
- Hypotension develops

- The QRS widens by 50% of its original width
- A total dose of 17 mg/kg has been given

Adverse Reactions/Side Effects: confusion, seizures, hypotension, ventricular arrhythmias, heart block, asystole.

Sodium Bicarbonate

Action: systemic hydrogen ion buffer, aids in the correction of metabolic acidosis.

Use: management of metabolic acidosis during cardiac arrest after the following:
- Prompt defibrillation
- Effective chest compressions
- ET intubation and hyperventilation using 100% oxygen
- Administration of at least two trials of epinephrine

Contraindications: none, when used in the treatment of metabolic acidosis.

Route/Dosage: 1 mEq/kg IVP initially. Repeat at 0.5 mEq/kg q 10 min during arrest if ventilation is adequate.

Adverse Reactions/Side Effects: fluid retention, metabolic alkalosis, hypokalemia, hypocalcemia.

Sodium Nitrite

Action: cyanide poisoning adjunct, degrades cyanide.

Use: second of a three-step treatment for cyanide poisoning, should be preceded by amyl nitrite and followed by sodium thiosulfate.

Contraindications: none.

Route/Dosage: 300 mg (one 10 mL ampule of a 3% sol) slow IVP (over 5 min) after amyl nitrite inhalation. Can also dilute 300 mg in 50–100 mL of NS and infuse slowly.

Adverse Reactions/Side Effects: hypotension, tachycardia, fainting.

Sodium Thiosulfate

Action: cyanide poisoning adjunct; detoxifies the body in cases of cyanide poisoning.

Use: third in a three-step treatment protocol for cyanide poisoning; preceded by amyl nitrite and sodium nitrite.

Contraindications: none.

Route/Dosage: 12.5 mL slow IVP (50 mL ampule of a 25% sol).

Adverse Reactions/Side Effects: none.

Streptokinase (Kabikinase, Streptase)

Action: thrombolytic; dissolves thrombi or emboli, preserving left ventricular function after MI.

Use treatment of the following:
- Coronary thrombosis associated with MI
- Pulmonary emboli

Contraindications: active internal bleeding, CVA within 2 mo, uncontrolled severe hypertension.

Route/Dosage: 1,500,000 International Units (IU) IV infusion over 60 min.

Adverse Reactions/Side Effects: bronchospasm, arrhythmias due to reperfusion, anaphylaxis.

Succinylcholine (Anectine, Quelicin, Sucostrin)

Action: skeletal muscle relaxant; causes skeletal muscle relaxation to aid in ET intubation.

Use: rapid skeletal muscle relaxation to assist in ET intubation.

Contraindications: narrow-angle glaucoma, penetrating eye injuries.

Route/Dosage: 1–2 mg/kg IVP. Can be repeated if necessary.

Adverse Reactions/Side Effects: respiratory depression, apnea, wheezing, arrhythmias, sinus arrest, hypertension, hypotension, increased intraocular pressure.

Syrup of Ipecac

Action: emetic; causes vomiting.

Use: inducement of vomiting in cases of poisoning or overdose in the alert patient.

Contraindications: reduced levels of consciousness, lost gag reflex, seizures, patients who have ingested caustic or petroleum products.

Route/Dosage: 15–30 mL PO, followed by several glasses of warm water.

Adverse Reactions/Side Effects: arrhythmias, hypotension, diarrhea.

Thiamine—Vitamin B_1 (Betalin S)

Action: B-complex vitamin; restores the body's supply of the vitamin.

Use: treatment of the following:
- Coma of unknown origin
- Coma due to alcohol
- Delirium tremens

Contraindications: none.
Route/Dosage: after giving $D_{50}W$,
- dilute 100 mg in 50–100 mL of NS or D_5W and infuse over 15–20 min.
- give 50 mg slow IVP and 50 mg IM.

Adverse Reactions/Side Effects: hypotension, dyspnea, respiratory failure.

Vecuronium (Norcuron)

Action: paralytic; skeletal muscle paralysis.
Use: inducement of skeletal muscle paralysis and facilitation of ET intubation.
Contraindications: neonates.
Route/Dosage: 80–100 µg/kg IVP.
Adverse Reactions/Side Effects: respiratory insufficiency, muscle weakness.

Verapamil (Calan, Isoptin)

Action: antianginal, antiarrhythmic, antihypertensive; decreases vascular resistance and reduces myocardial oxygen consumption.
Use: treatment of the following:
- PSVT
- Atrial fibrillation (rapid ventricular response)

Contraindications: sinus bradycardia, severe CHF, high-degree heart block, Wolff-Parkinson-White syndrome.
Route/Dosage: 2.5–5 mg IV over 5 min. Can repeat at 5–10 mg IV over 5 min q 15–30 min if needed.
Adverse Reactions/Side Effects: sinus arrest, asystole, heart block, bradycardia, hypotension, pulmonary edema.

TABLE 1. Glasgow Coma Scale for Adults

Eye Opening

  Spontaneously 4

  To command 3

  To pain 2

  No response 1

Verbal Response

  Oriented 5

  Confused 4

  Inappropriate words 3

  Incomprehensible 2

  No response . . . . .1 _____

Motor Response

  Obeys commands 6

  Localizes pain .5

  Withdraws from pain 4

  Flexion (decorticate) 3

  Extension (decerebrate) 2

  No response . . . . .1 _____

            Total:

PART II: PEDIATRICS

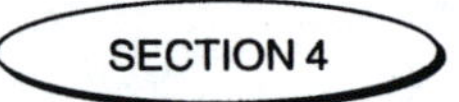

American Heart Association Treatment Algorithms

Bradycardia Decision Tree

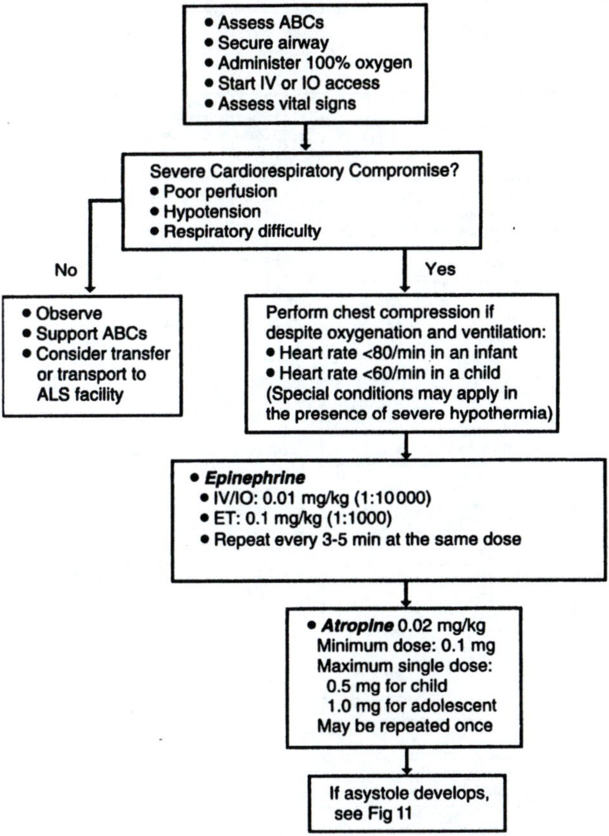

Figure 10. Bradycardia decision tree. ABCs indicate airway, breathing, and circulation; ALS, advanced life support; ET, endotracheal; IO, intraosseous; and IV, intravenous. (Reproduced with permission from Guidelines for Cardiopulmonary Resuscitation and Emergency Cardiac Care. Recommendations of the 1992 National Conference. American Heart Association. JAMA 268(16):2171–2302, October 28, 1992. Copyright 1992, American Medical Association.)

Asystole and Pulseless Arrest

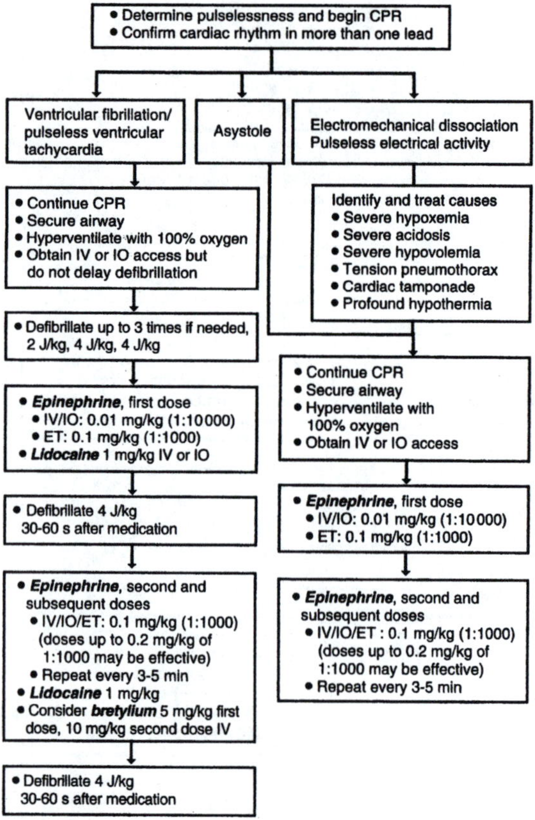

Figure 11. Asystole and pulseless arrest decision tree. CPR indicates cardiopulmonary resuscitation; ET, endotracheal; IO, intraosseous; and IV, intravenous. (Reproduced with permission from Guidelines for Cardiopulmonary Resuscitation and Emergency Cardiac Care. Recommendations of the 1992 National Conference. American Heart Association. JAMA 268(16):2171–2302, October 28, 1992. Copyright 1992, American Medical Association.)

TABLE 2. Statistically Common Pediatric Normal Values

Age	Average Weight*	Respiratory Rate (breaths/min)	Pulse Rate (beats/min)	Blood Pressure (mm Hg)†
Birth–6 weeks	4–5 kg (9–11 lb)	30–50	120–160	74–100 50–68
7 weeks–1 year	4–11 kg (9–24 lb)	20–30	80–140	84–106 45–70
1–2 years	11–14 kg (24–31 lb)	20–30	80–130	98–106 58–70
2–6 years	14–25 kg (31–55 lb)	20–30	80–120	98–112 64–70
6–13 years	25–63 kg (55–139 lb)	12–20	60–100	104–124 64–80
13–16 years	62–80 kg (136–176 lb)	12–20	60–100	118–132 70–82

*Weight estimation: $8 + (12 \times$ age [y]$) =$ weight in kg.
†Systolic blood pressure estimation: $80 + (2 \times$ age [y]$) =$ approx. systolic BP.
Source: Beck, RK: Pharmacology for Prehospital Emergency Care, ed. 2. F.A. Davis, Philadelphia, 1994, p 260.

TABLE 3. Drugs Used in Pediatric Advanced Life Support*

Drug	Dose	Remarks
Adenosine	0.1 to 0.2 mg/kg	Rapid IV bolus Maximum single dose: 12 mg
Atropine sulfate	0.02 mg/kg per dose	Minimum dose: 0.1 mg Maximum single dose: 0.5 mg in child, 1.0 mg in adolescent
Bretylium	5 mg/kg; may be increased to 10 mg/kg	Rapid IV
Calcium chloride 10%	20 mg/kg per dose	Give slowly
Dopamine hydrochloride	2–20 µg/kg/min	α-Adrenergic action dominates at $\geq$ 15–20 µg/kg/min
Dobutamine hydrochloride	2–20 µg/kg/min	Titrate to desired effect
Epinephrine for bradycardia	IV/IO; 0.01 mg/kg (1:10,000) ET: 0.1 mg/kg (1:1000)	Be aware of effective dose of high preservatives administered (if preservatives are present in epinephrine preparation) when doses are used

For asystolic or pulseless arrest	First dose:	Be aware of effective dose of preservative administered (if preservatives present in epinephrine preparation) when high doses are used
	IV/IO: 0.01 mg/kg (1:10,000)	
	ET: 0.1 mg/kg (1:1000)	
	Doses as high as 0.2 mg/kg may be effective	
	Subsequent doses:	
	IV/IO/ET: 0.1 mg/kg (1:1000)	
	Doses as high as 0.2 mg/kg may be effective	
Epinephrine infusion	Initial at 0.1 µg/kg/min	Titrate to desired effect (0.1–1.0 µg/kg/min)
	Higher infusion dose used if asystole present	
Lidocaine	1 mg/kg per dose	
Lidocaine infusion	20–50 µg/kg/min	
Sodium bicarbonate	1 mEq/kg per dose or $0.3 \times kg \times$ base deficit	Infuse slowly and only if ventilation is adequate

*IV indicates intravenous route: IO, intraosseous route; and ET, endotracheal route.
Source: Beck, RK: Pharmacology for Prehospital Emergency Care, ed. 2. F.A. Davis, Philadelphia, 1994, p 264.

Other Pediatric Medications

Activated Charcoal (Arm-a-char; Charcoaide, InstaChar): 10–30 g (3–5 tbs) mixed with water.

Albuterol (Proventil, Ventolin): > 12 years old—2 inhalations q 4–6 h (90 μg/spray). Do not use for patients under 12 years.

Aminophylline (Aminophyllin, Somophyllin): 6 mg/kg IV infusion over 20–30 min.

Amyl nitrite: 1 ampule crushed and inhaled for 30 sec. Repeat as needed.

Atropine for organophosphate poisoning: 0.05 mg/kg IVP. May repeat as needed.

Chlorpromazine (Promapan, Thorazine): 0.55 mg/kg IM.

Dextrose 50% in water/$D_{50}W$: 0.5–1.0 g/kg slow IVP of a 25% sol.

Diazepam (Valium, Valrelease):
- Seizures: 0.2–0.5 mg/kg IVP over 3 min
- Status epilepticus: < 5 years—0.2–0.5 mg IVP or IM (5 mg max.)
  > 5 years—1 mg q 2–5 min IVP or IM (10 mg max.)

Diazoxide (Hyperstat, Proglycem): 1–3 mg/kg IVP up to 150 mg.

Diphenhydramine (Benadryl, Benylin): 2–5 mg/kg slow IVP or deep IM.

Epinephrine (Adrenalin):
- Anaphylaxis: Mild/moderate: 0.01 mL/kg SC (1:1000 sol).
- Severe: 0.1 mL/kg IVP (1:10,000 sol).
- Bronchial asthma: 0.01 mL/kg SC (1:1000 sol). Do not exceed 0.5 mL in a single dose.

Hydrocortisone (Cortef, Cortisol, Hydrocortone, Solu-Cortef): 0.16–1.0 mg/kg IVP or IM.

Hydroxyzine (Atarax, Vistaril): 1.1 mg/kg deep IM.

Insulin (Humulin, Iletin, Novolin):
- IV: 0.1 U/kg IV bolus followed by IV infusion of 0.1 U/kg/h
- IV, SC: 0.5–1 U divided into 2; give 1/2 dose by IV bolus and 1/2 dose SC

Meperidine (Demerol): 1.1–1.8 mg/kg IM. Maximum dose = 100 mg.

Metaproterenol (Alupent, Metaprel): > 12 years—2 inhalations q 4–6 h (200 μg/spray).

Naloxone (Narcan): 0.01 mg/kg slow IVP.

Phenobarbital (Luminal):
- Anticonvulsant: 10–20 mg/kg slow IVP
- Status epilepticus: 15–20 mg/kg slow IVP

Phenytoin (Dilantin): 10–15 mg/kg slow IVP (0.5–1.5 mg/kg/min).

Physostigmine (Antilirium): 0.02 mg/kg slow IVP or IM.

Pralidoxime (Protopam): 20–40 mg/kg IV infusion over 30–60 min.

Propranolol (Inderal): 0.01 mg/kg slow IVP.

Racemic Epinephrine (Micro Nefrin):
- < 20 kg: 0.25 mL/kg by inhalation
- 20–40 kg: 0.5 mL/kg by inhalation

Sodium Nitrite: 0.15–0.33 mL/kg slow IVP.

Sodium Thiosulfate: 1.65 mL/kg of a 25% sol slow IVP.

Syrup of Ipecac:
- 6 months–1 year: 5–10 mL PO followed by water/juice
- > 1 year: 15–25 mL PO followed by water/juice

Terbutaline (Brethaire, Brethine, Bricanyl): >12 years old—2 inhalations q 4–6 h (200 µg/spray).

TABLE 4. Calculating Drug Concentrations and Infusion Rates for Common Pediatric Medications

Drug	Commonly Found Drug Concentration	Desired Rate of Administration (μg/kg/min)	Amount of Drug Solution to Add to 100 mL of D_5W (mL)
Isoproterenol	0.2 mg/mL	0.1	3
Epinephrine	1:1000 (1 mg/mL)	0.1	0.6
Dopamine	40 mg/mL	10	1.5
Dobutamine	25 mg/mL	10	2.4
Lidocaine	1% (10 mg/mL)	20	12

Listed above are five prehospital pediatric drugs. The chart shows, for each drug, the drug's concentration in its most common preparation and the rate of administration that medical control usually orders for the drug. The last column shows the amount of drug preparation to add to 100 mL of D_5W. By infusing the resulting solution at the rate of administration indicated on the body weight chart below, you will achieve the desired rate of drug administration.

WEIGHT		Infusion Rate (mL/h)	WEIGHT		Infusion Rate (mL/h)
kg	lb		kg	lb	
3	6.6	3	30	66	30
7	15.4	7	35	77	35
10	22	10	40	88	40
12.5	27.5	12.5	45	99	45
15	33	15	55	110	50
17.5	38.5	17.5	55	121	55
20	44	20	60	132	60
22.5	49.5	22.5	65	143	65
25	55	25	70	154	70

Source: Beck, RK: Pharmacology for Prehospital Emergency Care, ed. 2. F.A. Davis, Philadelphia, 1994, p 263.

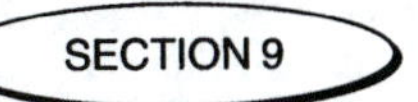

Intraosseous Infusion

Intraosseous infusion allows rapid vascular access via the bone marrow. It is used mostly to give fluids and drugs to children under 6 years who are suffering circulatory failure or cardiac arrest. Consult your local protocols as to age group and indications for using the IO procedure.

- Proximal tibia (preferred site): The needle will enter 1–3 cm below the tibial tuberosity just beneath the knee.
- Distal femur: The needle will enter 3 cm above the lateral condyle just above the knee.
- Distal tibia: The needle will enter in the flat surface of the tibia 1–3 cm above the medial malleolus at the ankle.

Preferred Site for Intraosseous
Drug Administration (Proximal Tibia)

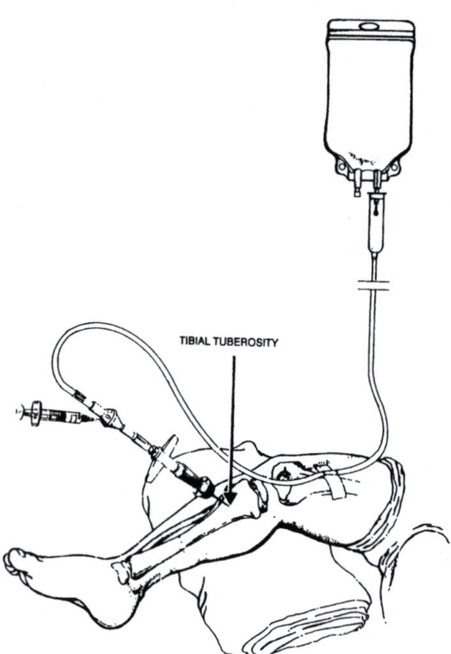

Figure 12. Preferred site for intraosseous drug administration (proximal tibia). (From Beck, RK: Pharmacology for Prehospital Emergency Care, ed. 2. F.A. Davis, Philadelphia, 1994, p 56.)

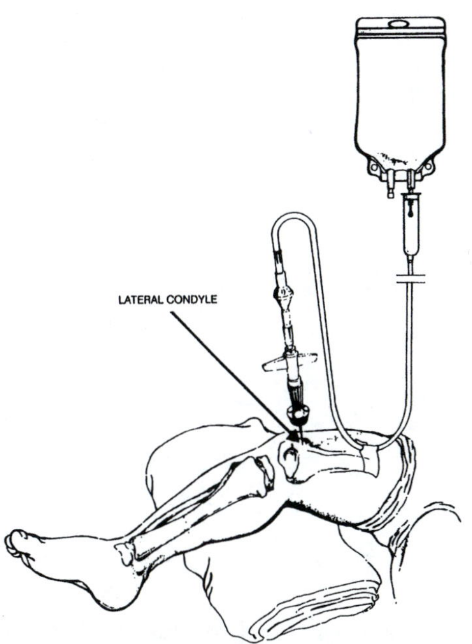

Figure 13. Intraosseous drug administration (distal femur). (From Beck, RK: Pharmacology for Prehospital Emergency Care, ed. 2. F.A. Davis, Philadelphia, 1994, p 56.)

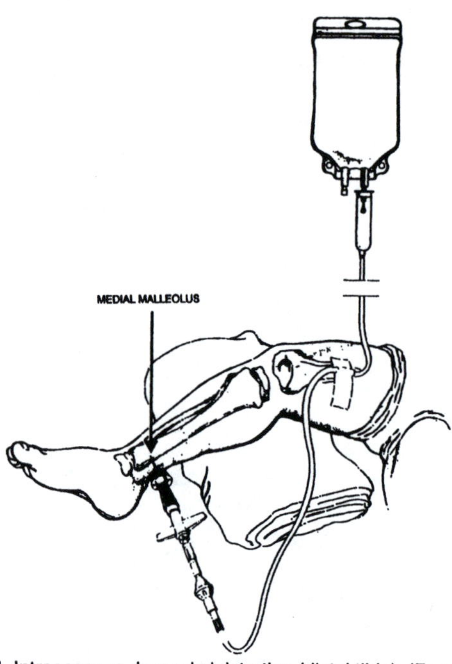

Figure 14. Intraosseous drug administration (distal tibia). (From Beck, RK: Pharmacology for Prehospital Emergency Care, ed. 2. F.A. Davis, Philadelphia, 1994, p 57.)

TABLE 5. Guidelines for Pediatric ET Tube and Suction Catheter Size

Patient Age	ET Tube Size (I.D. in mm)	Suction Catheter (F)
Premature	2.5–3.0 (uncuffed)	5–6
Term	3.0–3.5 (uncuffed)	6–8
6 months	3.5–4.0 (uncuffed)	8
1 year	4.0–4.5 (uncuffed)	8
2 years	4.5–5.0 (uncuffed)	8
4 years	5.0–5.5 (uncuffed)	10
6 years	5.5 (uncuffed)	10
8 years	6.0 (cuffed or uncuffed)	10
10 years	6.5 (cuffed or uncuffed)	12
12 years	7.0 (cuffed)	12

TABLE 6. Modified Glasgow Coma Scale for Infants and Children

	Infant	Score*	Child	Score*
Eye opening				
	Spontaneous	4	Spontaneous	4
	In response to verbal stimuli	3	In response to verbal stimuli	3
	In response to pain only	2	In response to pain only	2
	No response	1	No response	1
Verbal response				
	Coos, babbles	5	Oriented, appropriate	5
	Irritable cries	4	Confused	4
	Cries in response to pain	3	Inappropriate words	3
	Moans in response to pain	2	Nonspecific words/sounds	2
	No response	1	No response	1
Motor response				
	Normal movements	6	Obeys commands	6
	Withdraws in response to touch	5	Localizes painful stimulus	5
	Withdraws in response to pain	4	Withdraws in response to pain	4
	Abnormal flexion	3	Flexion in response to pain	3
	Abnormal extension	2	Extension in response to pain	2
	No response	1	No response	1

*Best possible score = 15; lowest possible score = 3.

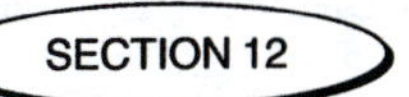

Newborn Resuscitation

The relative priorities of newborn resuscitation are as follows:
1. Dry, warm, position, suction, stimulate
2. Provide oxygen
3. Establish effective ventilation: 40–60/min when performed without compression
   - Bag-valve mask
   - Endotracheal intubation:

Weight (kg)	ET Tube Size (mm)	Catheter Size (F)
1	2.5	5
2	3.0	6
3	3.5	8
4	3.5	8

4. Chest compressions: 120/min (performed with ventilations)
   Compression: ventilation ratio: 3:1 (pause for ventilation)
5. Medications: Indicated if the heart remains <80 beats/min despite adequate ventilations with 100% oxygen and effective chest compressions.

Drug	Dose/Route
Epinephrine (1:10,000 sol)	0.01–0.03 mg/kg IV or ET
Naloxone	0.1 mg/kg IV, IM, SC, ET
Volume expanders:	
· 5% albumin	10 mL/kg IV
· Blood	10 mL/kg IV
· NS	10 mL/kg IV
· LR	10 mL/kg IV

Term newborn vital signs during first 12 hours of life:
- Heart rate: 100–180 beats/min
- Respirations: 30–60/min
- Blood pressure: 39–59/16–36 mm Hg

TABLE 7. Apgar Score

Sign	0	1	2
Heart rate/min	Absent	<100	>100
Respirations	Absent	Slow, irregular	Good, crying
Muscle tone	Limp	Some flexion	Active
Reflex irritability (catheter in nares)	No response	Grimace	Cough or sneeze
Color	Blue/pale	Pink body, extremities blue	Completely pink

Note: Apgar scores should be assessed at 1 and 5 minutes of age. If there is a score of < 7 at 5 minutes, additional scores should be obtained q 5 minutes for 20 minutes. The Apgar score should not be used to determine the need for resuscitation.

13

PART III: GENERAL

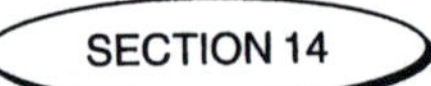

Drug-Dose Calculations

Metric-to-Metric Conversion

To go from larger measurements to a smaller measurement (grams to milligrams, or milligrams to micrograms) multiply by 1000 or move the decimal point three places to the right.

EXAMPLE: Convert 4 grams to milligrams: $4.0\,g \times 1000 = 4000\,mg$
EXAMPLE: Convert 1.5 L to milliliters: $1.5 \times 1000 = 1500\,mL$
EXAMPLE: Convert 5 milligrams to micrograms: $5 \times 1000 = 5000\,\mu g$

To go from a smaller measurement to a larger measurement, (milligrams to grams, or micrograms to milligrams) divide by 1000, or move the decimal point three places to the left.

EXAMPLE: Convert 3500 milligrams to grams: 3500 mg ÷ 1000 = 3.5 g
EXAMPLE: Convert 3000 milliliters to liters: 3000 mL ÷ 1000 = 3 L
EXAMPLE: Convert 50 micrograms to milligrams: 50 µg ÷ 1000 = 0.05 mg

Note that conversion to other metric units may require you to multiply or divide by some other factor of 10, as shown in Section 17.

Conversion of Pounds to Kilograms

To convert pounds to kilograms, divide the number of pounds by 2.2.

EXAMPLE: 100 lb ÷ 2.2 = 45 kg (45.45 is rounded down to 45)
EXAMPLE: 150 lb ÷ 2.2 = 68 kg (68.18 is rounded down to 68)

Calculation of Drug Solutions

To calculate drug concentration (mg/mL):

$$\text{Concentration} = \frac{\text{Amount of Drug (mg)}}{\text{Volume of Solution (mL)}}$$

EXAMPLE:

$$\text{Concentration} = \frac{500 \text{ mg (Total mg)}}{10 \text{ mL (Total mL)}} = 50 \text{ mg/mL}$$

To calculate how much solution (volume of drug) is required to deliver the amount of drug ordered:

$$\text{Required Volume of Solution (mL)} = \frac{\text{Required Drug Amount (mg)}}{\text{Drug Concentration (mg/mL)}}$$

EXAMPLE: Order = give 200 mg of a drug that has a concentration of 50 mg/mL. How much of the drug will be required to equal 200 mg?

$$\text{Required Volume of Solution (mL)} = \frac{200 \text{ mg}}{50 \text{ mg/mL}} = 4 \text{ mL}$$

Calculation of Rates of Infusion

$$\text{Infusion Rate (gtt/min)} = \frac{\text{Volume Required (mL)} \times \text{IV Set Size}}{\text{Infusion Time (min)}}$$

EXAMPLE:

$$\text{gtt/min} = \frac{500 \text{ mL} \times 15 \text{ gtt/mL}}{45 \text{ min}} = 167 \text{ gtt/min}$$

Conversion of Temperature Measurement

Degrees Celsius = (Degrees Fahrenheit − 32) × 0.556
Degrees Fahrenheit = Degrees Celsius × 1.8 + 32

Temperature Conversion

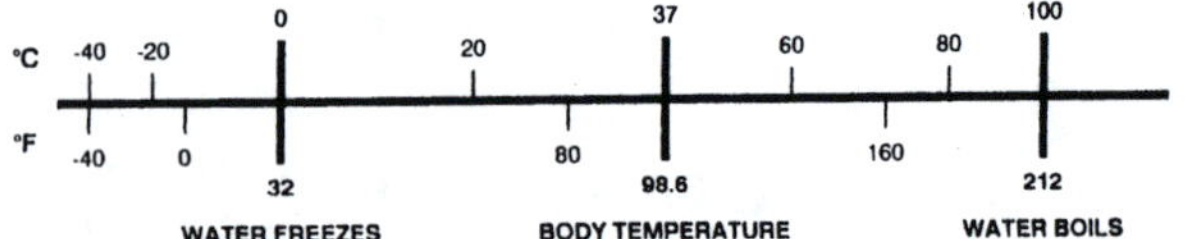

Figure 15. How the Fahrenheit and Celsius temperature scales compare. (From Beck, RK: Pharmacology for Prehospital Emergency Care, ed. 2. F.A. Davis, Philadelphia, 1994, p 73.)

SECTION 16

TABLE 8. Metric Conversion

Scale	Multiple of Base	Table	Grams
Mega	1,000,000	1 megagram	1,000,000.0
Kilo	1000	1 kilogram	1000.0
Hecto	100	1 hectogram	100.0
Deca	10	1 decagram	10.0
Base	1	1 gram	1.0
Deci	1/10	1 decigram	0.1
Centi	1/100	1 centigram	0.01
Milli	1/1000	1 milligram	0.001
Micro	1/1,000,000	1 microgram	10^{-6}

Commonly Used Equivalents

1 qt = 946 mL

1 fl oz = 30 mL

1 tbsp = 15 mL

1 tsp = 5 mL

1 kilogram (kg) = 2.2 pounds (lb)

0.454 kilograms (kg) = 1 pound (lb)

1 gram (g) = 0.035 ounces (oz)

28.35 grams (g) = 1 ounce (oz)

1 milligram (mg) = 0.015 grains

1 liter (L) = 1.057 quarts (qt)

TEMPERATURE		WEIGHT	
°F	°C	lb	kg
106	41.1	396	180
105	40.6	385	175
104	40.0	374	170
103	39.4	363	165
102	38.9	352	160
101	38.3	341	155
100	37.8	330	150

Table continued on following page

TABLE 8. (Continued)

TEMPERATURE		WEIGHT	
°F	°C	lb	kg
99	37.2	319	145
98.6	37.0	308	140
98	36.7	297	135
97	36.1	286	130
96	35.6	275	125
95	35.0	264	120
94	34.4	253	115
93	33.9	242	110
92	33.3	231	105
91	32.8	220	100
90	32.2	209	95
89	31.7	198	90
88	31.1	187	85
87	30.6	176	80
86	30.0	165	75
85	29.4	154	70
84	28.9	143	65
83	28.3	132	60
82	27.8	121	55
81	27.2	110	50
80	26.7	99	45

Common Abbreviations and Symbols

17

Abbreviation	Meaning
a.c.	before meals
admin.	administer, administration
ALS	advanced life support
AMI	acute myocardial infarction
amp.	ampule
amt.	amount
AV	atrioventricular
bid	twice a day
BP	blood pressure
c̄	with
caps	capsule
CHF	congestive heart failure
CNS	central nervous system
COPD	chronic obstructive pulmonary disease
CVA	cerebrovascular accident
CPR	cardiopulmonary resuscitation
d.	daily
D/C	discontinue
dig.	digitalis
dL	deciliter
Dx	diagnosis
ECC	emergency cardiac care
ECG/EKG	electrocardiogram
EGTA	esophageal gastric airway
EMS	emergency medical services
EOA	esophageal obturator airway
et	and
ETOH	ethyl alcohol
ETT	endotracheal tube
°F	degrees Fahrenheit

g or gm	gram
gr	grain
gtt(s)	drop(s)
h or hr	hour
Hx	history
IM	intramuscular
IO	intraosseous
IU	international unit
IV	intravenous
IVP	intravenous path
K	potassium ion
kg	kilogram
KO	keep open
KVO	keep vein open
L	left, liter
lb	pound
m	meter
mEq	milliequivalent
mg	milligram
MI	myocardial infraction
min	minutes
μg	microgram
mL	milliliter
mm	millimeter
MS or MSO_4	morphine sulfate
NA^+	sodium ion
$NaHCO_3$	sodium Bicarbonate
ng tube	nasogastric tube
nitro or NTG	nitroglycerin
NKA	no known allergies
NPO	nothing by mouth
NS	normal saline
OD	overdose
p.c.	after meals
P_{CO_2}	carbon dioxide pressure
PEA	pulseless electrical activity
Peds	pediatric
PO	by mouth
pH	hydrogen ion concentration

pO_2	oxygen pressure or tension
PR, pr	per rectum
prep	preparation
prm	as needed
PSVT	paroxysmal supraventricular tachycardia
q	every
qd	every day
qh	every hour
qid	four times a day
R	right
Rx	take; treatment
s̄	without
SC or SQ	subcutaneous
SL	sublingual
SOB	shortness of breath
sol	solution
ss	half
s/s	signs/symptoms
stat	at once
tab	tablet
tid	three times a day
TKO	to keep open
tbs	tablespoon
TBSA	total body surface area
U, u	unit
VE	ventricular fibrillation
VT	ventricular tachycardia
VO	verbal order
vol	volume
WNL	within normal limits
wt	weight
y.o.	year old
yr	year
↑	increase
↓	decrease
Ø	none
≈	approximate
♂	male
♀	female

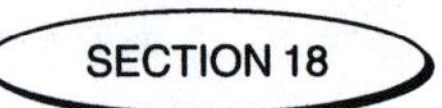

Rapid-Sequence Intubation

- Allow the patient to breathe 100% humidified oxygen by mask or assist ventilations as appropriate.
- Ensure that the patient has a functioning IV line in place.
- Ensure that the patient is connected to a cardiac monitor.
- Premedicate as follows:
  - Diazepam: 3–5 mg slow IVP. This is given for sedation of conscious patients.
  - Atropine: 0.01–0.02 mg/kg by IVP. This is for control of possible bradycardia, which may develop as a result of vagal stimulation during intubation in *pediatric* patients.
  - Lidocaine: 1 mg/kg IVP. This is given for intracranial pressure control in head-injured patients with central nervous system (CNS) injury.
  - Succinylcholine: 1–2 mg/kg IVP.
- Proceed with intubation.

Common Laboratory Values

Blood

Hematocrit (Hct)

Men	42–52%
Women	37–47% (pregnancy: >33%)
Children	31–43%
Infants	30–40%
Newborns	44–64%

Hemoglobin (Hgb)

Men	14–18 g/dL
Women	12–16 g/dL (pregnancy: >11 g/dL)
Children	11–16 g/dL
Infants	10–15 g/dL
Newborns	14–24 g/dL

Red Blood Count (RBC)

Men	4.7–6.1 million/mm^3
Women	4.2–5.4 million/mm^3
Infants and children	3.8–5.5 million/mm^3
Newborns	4.8–7.1 million/mm^3

White Blood Count (WBC)

Adults and children >2 years	5000–10,000/cm^3
Children <2 years	6200–17,000/mm^3
Newborns	9000–30,000/mm^3

Venereal Disease Research Laboratory (VDRL)	**Negative**

Glucose, Fasting (FBS)

Adults	70–115 mg/dL
Children	60–100 mg/dL
Newborns	30–80 mg/dL

Electrolytes

Sodium	136–145 mEq/L
Potassium	3.5–5.5 mEq/L
Magnesium	1.6–3.0 mEq/L
Calcium	10.5–11 mg or 4.3–5.3 mEq/L
Chloride	95–108 mEq/L
Blood urea nitrogen (BUN)	5–20 mg/dL
Cholesterol	150–250 mg/dL

Urine

Color	Straw color
RBC	Neg. or 0
WBC	Neg. or 0
pH	4.8–8.0
Specific gravity	1.010–1.030
Bacteria	Neg. or 0
Glucose	Neg. or 0
Acetone	Neg. or 0
Albumin (protein)	Neg. or 0

Blood Gases

PO_2	80–100 mm Hg
PCO_2	35–45 mm Hg
HCO_3	22–26 mEq
pH (arterial)	7.35–7.45
Bilirubin (total)	0.1–1.2 mg
O_2 sat (arterial)	95% or greater
Base excess (BE)	–2 to +2

Note: Normal laboratory values may vary, depending on the methods used to determine the values.

TABLE 9. IV Solutions

Solution	Indications	Contraindications
Colloids		
Plasma protein fraction	Hypovolemic shock	None
Dextran	Hypovolemic shock	Known hypersensitivity
		Patient receiving anticoagulants
Hetastarch	Hypovolemic shock	None
Crystalloids		
Lactated Ringer's (LR)	Hypovolemic shock	CHF, renal failure
	IV drug route	
Dextrose 5% in water (D_5W)	IV drug route Dilution for concentrated drugs for IV infusion	Volume replacement
Dextrose 10% in water ($D_{10}W$)	Hypoglycemia ETOH intoxication Neonatal resuscitations	Volume replacement
Normal saline (NS; 0.9% sodium chloride)	IV drug route Hypovolemia	CHF
	Heat-related emergencies	
	Freshwater drowning	
	Diabetic ketoacidosis (DKA)	
	Dilute/warm blood	

Table continued on following page

TABLE 9. (Continued)

Solution	Indications	Contraindications
	Mainline for blood transfusion	
1/2 Normal saline (1/2 NS; 0.45% sodium chloride)	Compromised cardiac function	Emergency rehydration
Dextrose 5% in 1/2 normal saline ($D_5$1/2NS)	Heat emergencies Diabetic emergencies	Emergency rehydration
Dextrose 5% in normal saline (D_5NS)	Heat emergencies Volume replacement Freshwater drowning	Compromised cardiac/ renal function
Dextrose 5% in lactated Ringer's (D_5LR)	Volume replacement	Compromised cardiac/ renal function

Burn Treatment

Parkland Formula for Resuscitation

Day 1:

4 mL × TBSA × Weight (kg) (Ringer's lactate)
Give 1/2 of total fluid in first 8 h.
Give remaining 1/2 of fluid over next 16 h.

Day 2:

0.5 mL colloid × TBSA × Weight (kg)
(5% albumin or plasmanate)
Plus: 2000 mL of D_5W (maintenance in pediatrics)
Run concurrently over 24 h.

EXAMPLE (day 1): Patient = 8 yr old weighing 55 lbs (25 kg) with 87% TBSA burned.

$$4 \times 87 \times 25 = 8700 \text{ mL}$$
$$\text{First } 8 \text{ h} = 4350 \text{ mL} = 544 \text{ mL/h}$$
$$\text{Next } 16 \text{ h} = 272 \text{ mL/h}$$

Criteria for Burn Center Referral

Must be as follows: (Follow local protocols)
1. Second- or third-degree burns
2. Greater than 10% TBSA in patients <10 yr old
3. Greater than 20% in other ages
4. Burns of face, hands, feet, perineum
5. Inhalation burn
6. Electrical or chemical burns

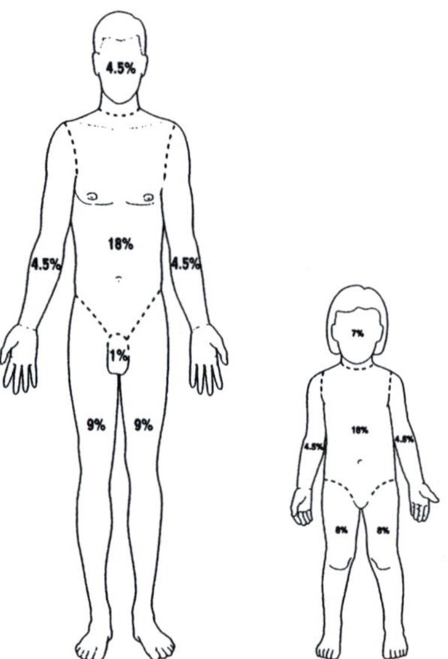

Figure 16. "Rule of nines" burn chart, adult and child body surface areas. (From Traynor, OT et al: The Streetmedic's Handbook. F. A. Davis, Philadelphia, 1996, pp 469–470.

TABLE 10. Dysrhythmia Recognition

	Rhythm	Rate	P Wave	QRS	PRI
Sinus Rhythms:					
Sinus rhythm	Regular	60–100	Upright	<0.10	0.12–0.20
Sinus bradycardia	Regular	<60	Upright	<0.10	0.12–0.20
Sinus tachycardia	Regular	>100	Upright	<0.10	0.12–0.20
Sinus arrhythmia	Irregular	Generally 60–100	Upright	<0.10	0.12–0.20
Atrial Rhythms:					
Supraventricular tachycardia (SVT)	Regular	160–250	Flattened or notched; may be lost in T wave	<0.10	<0.12 if seen
Atrial flutter	Regular or irregular	Atrial 250–350; ventricular variable	Flutter waves (sawtooth)	<0.10	Not measurable
Atrial fibrillation	Irregular	Atrial >400; ventricular variable	None	<0.10	Not measurable

Table continued on following page

75

22

TABLE 10. (Continued)

	Rhythm	Rate	P Wave	QRS	PRI
Junctional Rhythms:					
Junctional escape	Regular	40–60	Inverted, if seen; may occur before, during, or after QRS	<0.10	<0.12 if present
Accelerated	Regular	60–100	Inverted, if seen; may occur before, during, or after QRS	<0.10	<0.12 if present
Junctional tachycardia	Regular	100–180	Inverted if seen; may occur before, during, or after QRS	<0.10	<0.12 if present
Ventricular Rhythms:					
Agonal	Irregular	<20	Absent	>0.12	Not measurable
Idioventricular	Generally regular	20–40	Retrograde or absent; may appear after QRS; upright in ST segment or T wave	>0.12	Not measurable
Accelerated idioventricular	Generally regular	40–100	Retrograde or absent; may appear after QRS; upright in ST segment or T wave	>0.12	Not measurable

Ventricular tachycardia	Generally regular	>100	Retrograde or absent	>0.12	Not measurable
Torsades de pointes	Irregular	>150	None	>0.12	Not measurable
Ventricular fibrillation	Irregular/ chaotic	N/A	Absent	Absent	Absent
Asystole	None	N/A	None	None	None
AV Blocks:					
First Degree	Regular	Generally 60–100	Upright	<0.10	>0.20 constant
Second degree type 1 (Wenckebach)	Irregular	Generally 60–100	Upright; some are not followed by QRS	<0.10	Lengthens until P is not followed by QRS
Second degree type II	Irregular	Varies; atrial is more than ventricular	Upright; some are not followed by QRS	Generally >0.10	Normal/prolonged; constant for each conducted QRS
Third degree (complete)	regular	Varies; atrial is more than ventricular	More P waves than QRS complexes	<0.10 (junction) >0.10 (ventricles)	None

−90 to 180: Extreme right axis deviation—QRS negative in I and aVF.

0 to −90: Left axis deviation—QRS negative in a VF. QRS positive in I.

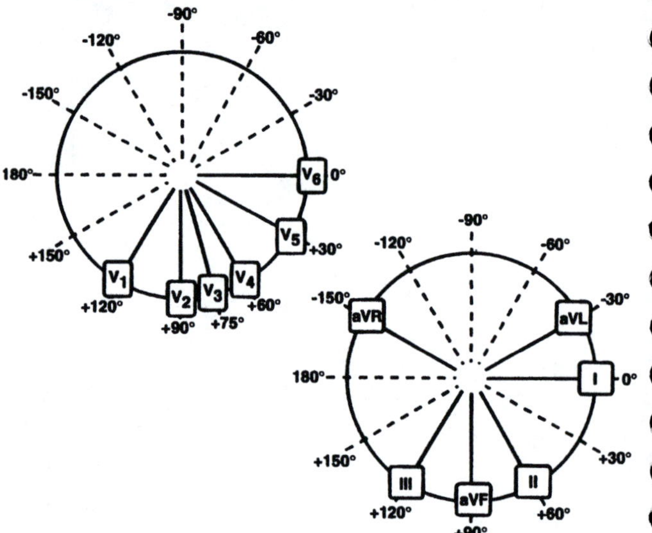

+90 to 180: Right axis deviation—QRS negative in I

0 to +90 Normal Range—Positive QRS in I and a VF.

Infarction Location (Left Ventricle)

Anterior: Q waves and ST elevation in V_1, V_2, V_3, or V_4
Lateral: Q waves in I and a VL
Inferior: Q waves and ST elevation in II, III, and a VF
Posterior: Large R wave and ST depression in V_1, Q wave in V_6. Try mirror test as follows: turn ECG upside down and look at V_1 and V_2 in a mirror. You should see signs of AMI: significant Q wave and ST elevation.

Figure 17. ECG axis.

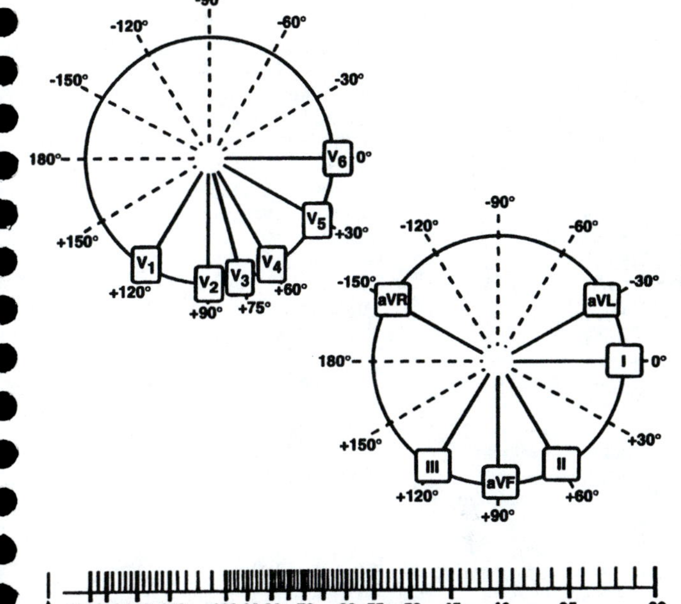

Figure 18. Heart rate at 25 mm/sec.

Common Medications

Drug Name	Therapeutic Classification(s)
A-MethaPred (methylprednisolone)	Anti-inflammatory, immunosuppressant
acebutolol	Antihypertensive, antiarrhythmic
Acephen (acetaminophen)	Non-narcotic analgesic, antipyretic
acetaminophen	Non-narcotic analgesic, antipyretic
acetazolamide	Anticonvulsant, diuretic
acetohexamide	Antidiabetic
acetophenazine	Antipsychotic
Activase (alteplase)	Antithrombolytic enzyme
Adalat (nifedipine)	Antianginal
Adapin (doxepin)	Antidepressant
Adrenalin Chloride (epinephrine hydrochloride)	Bronchodilator, vasopressor, cardiac stimulant, local anesthetic adjunct, topical antihemorrhagic, antiglaucoma agent
Aerolate (theophylline)	Bronchodilator
Akineton (biperidin)	Antiparkinsonian
Ak-Zol (acetazolamide)	Anticonvulsant, diuretic
Alazsine Tabs (hydralazine)	Antihypertensive
albuterol	Bronchodilator
Aldactone (spironolactone)	Antihypertensive, diuretic
Aldoclor (chlorothiazide/ methyldopa)	Diuretic, antihypertensive
Alphancaine (lidocaine)	Ventricular antiarrhythmic, local anesthetic
alprazolam	Antianxiety agent—controlled substance, Schedule IV

---

* Drug names beginning with a capital letter are trade; drug names beginning with a lowercase letter are generic.

Drug Name	Therapeutic Classification(s)
alteplase	Thrombolytic enzyme
Alupent (metaproterenol)	Bronchodilator
Alzapam (lorazepam)	Antianxiety agent, sedative/hypotic —controlled substance, Schedule IV
Amcill (ampicillin)	Antibiotic
A-methaPred (methylprednisolone)	Anti-inflammatory
Aminophyllin (aminophylline)	Bronchodilator
aminophylline	Bronchodilator
amiodarone	Ventricular and supraventricular antiarrhythmic
amitriptyline	Antidepressant
amobarbital	Sedative/hypnotic, anticonvulsant— controlled substance, Schedule II
Amodopa Tabs (methyldopa)	Antihypertensive
Amoline (aminophylline)	Bronchodilator
amoxapine	Antidepressant
amoxicillin	Antibiotic
Amoxil (amoxicillin)	Antibiotic
amphotericin B	Antifungal
ampicillin	Antibiotic
amrinone	inotropic, vasodilator
amyl nitrite	Cyanide poisoning adjunct
Amytal (amobarbital)	Sedative/hypnotic, anticonvulsant— controlled substance, Schedule II
Anacin-3 (acetaminophen)	Non-narcotic analgesic, antipyretic
Anestacon (lidocaine)	Ventricular antiarrhythmic, local anesthetic
Anspor (cephradine)	Antibiotic
Antilirium (physostigmine)	Antimuscarinic
Apo-Amitriptyline (amitriptyline)	Antidepressant
Apresoline (hydralazine)	Antihypertensive
Aprozide (hydrochlorothiazide)	Diuretic, antihypertensive

---

* Drug names beginning with a capital letter are trade; drug names beginning with a lowercase letter are generic.

Drug Name	Therapeutic Classification(s)
Aquachloral (chloral hydrate)	Sedative/hypnotic—controlled substance, Schedule IV
Aquatensen (methyclothiazide)	Diuretic, antihypertensive
Arm-a-Med (isoetharine)	Bronchodilator
Asendin (amoxapine)	Antidepressant
Asthma Nefrin (epinephrine hydrochloride)	Bronchodilator, vasopressor, cardiac stimulant, local anesthetic adjunct, topical antihemorrhagic, antiglaucoma agent
Asthmahaler (epinephrine bitartrate)	Bronchodilator, vasopressor, cardiac stimulant, local anesthetic adjunct, topical antihemorrhagic, antiglaucoma agent
Astramorph (morphine)	Analgesic—controlled substance, Schedule II
Atarax (hydroxyzine)	Antianxiety agent, sedative
atenolol	Antihypertensive, antianginal
atropine	Antiarrhythmic
Atrovent (ipratropium)	Bronchodilator
Aventyl (nortriptyline)	Antidepressant
bacampicillin	Antibiotic
Barbased (butabarbital)	Sedative/hypnotic—controlled substance, Schedule III
Barbita (phenobarbital)	Anticonvulsant, sedative/hypnotic—controlled substance, Schedule IV
beclomethasone	Anti-inflammatory, antiasthmatic
Beclovent (beclomethasone)	Anti-inflammatory, antiasthmatic
Beconase (beclomethasone)	Anti-inflammatory, antiasthmatic
Beef Regular Iletin II (insulin [regular])	Antidiabetic agent
Beldin (diphenhydramine)	Antihistamine, antiemetic and antivertigo agent, antitussive,

---

Drug Name	Therapeutic Classification(s)
	sedative/hypnotic, topical anesthetic
Benadryl (diphenhydramine)	Antihistamine, antiemetic and antivertigo agent, antitussive, sedative/hypnotic, topical anesthetic
Benadryl (diphenhydramine)	Antihistamine, antiemetic and antivertigo agent, antitussive, sedative/hypnotic, topical anesthetic
Benadryl Complete Allergy (diphenhydramine)	Antihistamine, antiemetic and antivertigo agent, antitussive, sedative/hypnotic, topical anesthetic
Bendylate (diphenhydramine)	Antihistamine, antiemetic and antivertigo agent, antitussive, sedative/hypnotic, topical anesthetic
Benylin (diphenhydramine)	Antihistamine, antiemetic and antivertigo agent, antitussive, sedative/hypnotic, topical anesthetic
Benylin DM Cough (dextromethorphan)	Non-narcotic antitussive
benzphetamine	Anorexigenic agent
biperidin	Antiparkinsonian
bitolterol	Bronchodilator
Blocadren (timolol)	Antihypertensive, antiglaucoma agent
Brethine (terbutaline)	Bronchodilator
bretylium tosylate	Antiarrhythmic
Bretylol (bretylium)	Antiarrhythmic
Bricanyl (terbutaline)	Bronchodilator
Bromo Seltzer (acetaminophen)	Non-narcotic analgesic, antipyretic
bromocriptine	Antiparkinsonian agent

Drug Name	Therapeutic Classification(s)
Bronitin Mist (epinephrine bitartrate)	Bronchodilator, vasopressor, cardiac stimulant, local anesthetic adjunct, topical antihemorrhagic, antiglaucoma agent
Bronkaid Mist (epinephrine)	Bronchodilator, vasopressor, cardiac stimulant, local anesthetic adjunct, topical antihemorrhagic, antiglaucoma agent
Bronkaid Mist Suspension (epinephrine bitartrate)	Bronchodilator, vasopressor, cardiac stimulant, local anesthetic adjunct, topical antihemorrhagic, antiglaucoma agent
Bronkodyl (theophylline)	Bronchodilator
Bronkosol (isoetharine)	Bronchodilator
Bumetanide	Antihypertensive, diuretic
Bumex (bumetanide)	Antihypertensive, diuretic
butabarbital	Sedative/hypnotic—controlled substance, Schedule III
Butalan (butabarbital)	Sedative/hypnotic—controlled substance, Schedule III
Buticaps (butabarbital)	Sedative/hypnotic—controlled substance, Schedule III
Butisol (butabarbital)	Sedative/hypnotic—controlled substance, Schedule III
butorphanol	Narcotic agonist-antagonist, opioid partial agonist
Calan (verapamil)	Antianginal, antiarrhythmic, antihypertensive
Capoten (captopril)	Antihypertensive
calcium chloride	Electrolyte modifier
calcium gluceptate	Electrolyte modifier
calcium gluconate	Electrolyte modifier
captopril	Antihypertensive
carbamazepine	Anticonvulsant, analgesic
carbenicillin	Antibiotic
Cardizem (diltiazem)	Antianginal
Catapres (clonidine)	Antihypertensive

* Drug names beginning with a capital letter are trade; drug names beginning with a lowercase letter are generic.

Drug Name	Therapeutic Classification(s)
Catapres-TTS (clonidine)	Antihypertensive
Ceclor (cefaclor)	Antibiotic
Cedilanid-D (deslanoside)	Antiarrhythmic, inotropic
cefaclor	Antibiotic
Celontin Half Strength Kapseals (methsuximide)	Anticonvulsant
Celontin Kapseals (methsuximide)	Anticonvulsant
Centrax (prazepam)	Antianxiety agent—controlled substance, Schedule IV
cephradine	Antibiotic
chloral hydrate	Sedative/hypnotic—controlled substance, Schedule IV
Chlorpazine (prochlorperazine)	Antipsychotic, antiemetic, antianxiety agent
chlordiazepoxide	Antianxiety agent, anticonvulsant, sedative/hypnotic—controlled substance, Schedule IV
chlorothiazide	Diuretic, antihypertensive
chlorpromazine	Antipsychotic, antiemetic
chlorpropamide	Antidiabetic, antidiuretic agent
chlorprothixene	Antipsychotic
chlorthalidone	Diuretic, antihypertensive
Choledyl (oxtriphylline)	Bronchodilator
Cin-Quin (quinidine)	Ventricular and supraventricular antiarrhythmic, atrial antiarrhythmic
clemastine	Antihistamine
clonazepam	Anticonvulsant—controlled substance, Schedule IV
clonidine	Antihypertensive
clorazepate	Antianxiety agent, anticonvulsant, sedative/hypnotic—controlled substance, Schedule IV
codeine	Analgesic, antitussive—controlled substance, Schedule II

23

---

* Drug names beginning with a capital letter are trade; drug names beginning with a lowercase letter are generic.

Drug Name	Therapeutic Classification(s)
Calan (verapamil)	Antianginal, antihypertensive, antiarrhythmic
Compazine (prochlorperazine)	Antipsychotic, antiemetic, antianxiety agent
Compazine Spansules (prochlorperazine)	Antipsychotic, antiemetic, antianxiety agent
Compo (diphenhydramine)	Antihistamine, antiemetic and antivertigo agent, antitussive, sedative/hypnotic, topical anesthetic
Congespzrin for children (dextromethorphan)	Non-narcotic antitussive
Constant-T (theophylline)	Bronchodilator
Cordarone (amiodarone)	Ventricular and supraventricular antiarrhythmic
Corgard (nadolol)	Antihypertensive, antianginal
Cortef (hydrocortisone)	Anti-inflammatory
Coumadin (warfarin)	Anticoagulant
Cremacoat 1 (dextromethorphan)	Non-narcotic antitussive
Crystodigin (digitoxin)	Antiarrhythmic agent, inotropic agent
Dalcaine (lidocaine)	Ventricular antiarrhythmic, local anesthetic
Dalmane (flurazepam)	Sedative/hypnotic—controlled substance, Schedule IV
Darvon (propoxyphene)	Analgesic—controlled substance, Schedule IV
Datril (acetaminophen)	Non-narcotic analgesic, antipyretic
Datril-500 (acetaminophen)	Non-narcotic analgesic, antipyretic
Decadron (dexamethasone)	Anti-inflammatory
Delsym (dextromethorphan)	Non-narcotic antitussive
Demerol (meperidine)	Analgesic—controlled substance, Schedule II

---

* Drug names beginning with a capital letter are trade; drug names beginning with a lowercase letter are generic.

Drug Name	Therapeutic Classification(s)
Depakene (valproic acid)	Anticonvulsant
Deprol (meprobamate)	Antianxiety agent—controlled substance, Schedule IV
desipramine	Antidepressant, antianxiety agent
deslanoside	Antiarrhythmic, inotropic
dexamethasone	Anti-inflammatory
dextromethorphan	Non-narcotic antitussive
dextrose 50% in water	Hyperglycemic
Dey-Dose (isoetharine)	Bronchodilator
Dey-Lute (isoetharine)	Bronchodilator
DiaBeta (glyburide)	Antidiabetic
Diabinese (chlorpropamide)	Antidiabetic, antidiuretic agent
Diaclor H (hydrochlorothiazide)	Diuretic, antihypertensive
Diahist (diphenhydramine)	Antihistamine, antiemetic and antivertigo agent, antitussive, sedative/hypnotic, topical anesthetic
Diamox (acetazolamide)	Anticonvulsant, diuretic
Diamox Sequels (acetazolamide)	Anticonvulsant, diuretic
diazepam	Antianxiety agent, skeletal muscle relaxant, amnesic agent, anticonvulsant, sedative/hypnotic
diazoxide	Antihypertensive
Didrex (benzphetamine)	Anorexigenic agent
digitoxin	Antiarrhythmic, inotropic
digoxin	Antiarrhythmic, inotropic
Dilantin (phenytoin)	Anticonvulsant, antiarrhythmic
Dilaudid (hydromorphone)	Analgesic, antitussive
Dilocaine (lidocaine)	Ventricular antiarrhythmic, local anesthetic
diltiazem	Antianginal
Diphen	Antihistamine, antiemetic and

23

---

* Drug names beginning with a capital letter are trade; drug names beginning with a lowercase letter are generic.

Drug Name	Therapeutic Classification(s)
(diphenhydramine)	antivertigo agent, antitussive, sedative/hypnotic, topical anesthetic
Diphenadryl (diphenhydramine)	Antihistamine, antiemetic and antivertigo agent, antitussive, sedative/hypnotic, topical anesthetic
diphenhydramine	Antihistamine, antiemetic and antivertigo agent, antitussive, sedative/hypnotic, topical anesthetic
dipyridamole	Coronary vasodilator, platelet aggregation inhibitor
disopyramide	Ventricular/supraventricular antiarrhythmia, atrial antitachyarrhythmic
Dispos-a-Med (isoetharine)	Bronchodilator
Diuril (chlorothiazide)	Diuretic, antihypertensive
DM Cough (dextromethorphan)	Non-narcotic antitussive
dobutamine	Inotropic
Dobutrex (dobutamine)	Inotropic
Dolene (propoxyphene)	Analgesic—controlled substance, Schedule IV
Dolophine (methadone)	Analgesic, narcotic detoxification adjunct—controlled substance, Schedule II
dopamine	Inotropic, vasopressor
Dopastat (dopamine)	Inotropic, vasopressor
Doriden (glutethimide)	Sedative/hypnotic—controlled substance, Schedule III
Doriglute (glutethimide)	Sedative/hypnotic—controlled substance, Schedule III
Doxaphene (propoxyphene)	Analgesic—controlled substance, Schedule IV

---

* Drug names beginning with a capital letter are trade; drug names beginning with a lowercase letter are generic.

Drug Name	Therapeutic Classification(s)
doxepin	Antidepressant
Duramorph (morphine)	Analgesic—controlled substance, Schedule II
Durapam (flurazepam)	Sedative/hypnotic—controlled substance, Schedule IV
Dymelor (acetohexamide)	Antidiabetic
Edecrin (ethacrynic acid)	Diuretic
edrophonium	Antiarrhythmic, cholinergic agonist
Elavil (amitriptyline)	Antidepressant
Elixophyllin (theophylline)	Bronchodilator
Emitrip (amitriptyline)	Antidepressant
Endep (amitriptyline)	Antidepressant
Enduron (methyclothiazide)	Diuretic, antihypertensive
Enovil (amitriptyline)	Antidepressant
Epifrin (epinephrine hydrochloride)	Bronchodilator, vasopressor, cardiac stimulant, local anesthetic adjunct, topical antihemorrhagic, antiglaucoma agent
epinephrine	Bronchodilator, vasopressor, cardiac stimulant, local anesthetic adjunct, topical antihemorrhagic, antiglaucoma agent
epinephrine bitartrate	Bronchodilator, vasopressor, cardiac stimulant, local anesthetic adjunct, topical antihemorrhagic, antiglaucoma agent
epinephrine hydrochloride	Bronchodilator, vasopressor, cardiac stimulant, local anesthetic adjunct, topical antihemorrhagic, antiglaucoma agent
EpiPen (epinephrine)	Bronchodilator, vasopressor, cardiac stimulant, local anesthetic adjunct, topical antihemorrhagic, antiglaucoma agent

* Drug names beginning with a capital letter are trade; drug names beginning with a lowercase letter are generic.

Drug Name	Therapeutic Classification(s)
EpiPen Jr. (epinephrine)	Bronchodilator, vasopressor, cardiac stimulant, local anesthetic adjunct, topical antihemorrhagic, antiglaucoma agent
Epitol (carbamazepine)	Anticonvulsant, analgesic
Epitrate (epinephrine bitartrate)	Bronchodilator, vasopressor, cardiac stimulant, local anesthetic adjunct, topical antihemorrhagic, antiglaucoma agent
Equanil (meprobarnate)	Antianxiety agent—controlled substance, Schedule IV
Esidrex (hydrochlorothiazide)	Diuretic, antihypertensive
Eskalith (lithium)	Antimanic, antipsychotic
Eskalith CR (lithium)	Antimanic, antipsychotic
ethacrynic acid	Diuretic
ethchlorvynol	Sedative/hypnotic—controlled substance, Schedule IV
ethosuximide	Anticonvulsant
Eutonyl (pargyline)	Antihypertensive
Extentabs (quinidine)	Ventricular and supraventricular antiarrhythmic, atrial antiarrhythmic
Fenylhist (diphenhydramine)	Antihistamine, antiemetic and antivertigo agent, antitussive, sedative/hypnotic, topical anesthetic
flecainide	Ventricular antiarrhythmic
flurazepam	Sedative/hypnotic—controlled substance, Schedule IV
Fungizone (amphotericin B)	Antifungal
furosemide	Diuretic, antihypertensive
Fynex (diphenhydramine)	Antihistamine, antiemetic and antivertigo agent, antitussive, sedative/hypnotic, topical anesthetic

* Drug names beginning with a capital letter are trade; drug names beginning with a lowercase letter are generic.

Drug Name	**Therapeutic Classification(s)**
Geocillin (carbenicillin)	Antibiotic
Glaucon (epinephrine hydrochloride)	Bronchodilator, vasopressor, cardiac stimulant, local anesthetic adjunct, topical antihemorrhagic, antiglaucoma agent
glipizide	Antidiabetic agent
Glucamide (chlorpropamide)	Antidiabetic, antidiuretic agent
Glucotrol (glipizide)	Antidiabetic agent
glutethimide	Sedative/hypnotic—controlled substance, Schedule III
glyburide	Antidiabetic
guanabenz	Antihypertensive
guanethidine	Antihypertensive
halazepam	Antianxiety agent—controlled substance, Schedule IV
Halcion (triazolam)	Sedative/hypnotic—controlled substance, Schedule III
Haldol (haloperidol)	Antipsychotic
haloperidol	Antipsychotic
Hexadrol (dexamethasone)	Anti-inflammatory
Hold (dextromethorphan)	Non-narcotic antitussive
Humulin R (insulin [regular])	Antidiabetic agent
hydralazine	Antihypertensive
Hydramine (diphenhydramine)	Antihistamine, antiemetic and antivertigo agent, antitussive, sedative/hypnotic, topical anesthetic
Hydra-Zide (hydrochlorothiazide)	Diuretic, antihypertensive
Hydril (diphenhydramine)	Antihistamine, antiemetic and antivertigo agent, antitussive, sedative/hypnotic, topical anesthetic
Hydro-DIURIL (hydrochlorothiazide)	Diuretic-antihypertensive

23

* Drug names beginning with a capital letter are trade; drug names beginning with a lowercase letter are generic.

Drug Name	**Therapeutic Classification(s)**
hydrochlorothiazide	Diuretic, antihypertensive
hydrocortisone	Anti-inflammatory
Hydrocortone (hydrocortisone)	Anti-inflammatory
hydromorphone	Analgesic, antitussive
hydroxyzine	Antianxiety agent, sedative
Hygroton (chlorthalidone)	Diuretic, antihypertensive
Hyperstat IV (diazoxide)	Antihypertensive
Inderal (propranolol)	Antihypertensive, antianginal, antiarrhythmic
Inderal LA (propranolol)	Antihypertensive, antianginal, antiarrhythmic
Inocor (amrinone)	Inotropic, vasodilator
insulin (regular)	Antidiabetic agent
Intropin (dopamine)	Inotropic, vasopressor
ipratropium	Bronchodilator
Ismelin (guanethidine)	Antihypertensive
isocarboxazid	Antidepressant
isocarboxazid	Antidepressant
isoetharine	Bronchodilator
isoproterenol	Antiarrhythmic, bronchodilator, cardiac stimulant
Isoptin (verapamil)	Antianginal, antihypertensive, antiarrhythmic
Isorbid (isosorbide dinitrate)	Antianginal, vasodilator
isosorbide	Antianginal, vasodilator
Klavikordal (nitroglycerin [oral])	Antianginal, vasodilator
Klonopin (clonazepam)	Anticonvulsant—controlled substance, Schedule IV
labetalol	Antihypertensive
Lanoxicaps (digoxin)	Antiarrhythmic agent, inotropic agent
Lanoxin (digoxin)	Antiarrhythmic, inotropic
Lasix (furosemide)	Diuretic, antihypertensive

---

* Drug names beginning with a capital letter are trade; drug names beginning with a lowercase letter are generic.

Drug Name	Therapeutic Classification(s)
L-Caine (lidocaine)	Ventricular antiarrhythmic, local anesthetic
Levoprome (methotrimeprazine)	Sedative, analgesic agent, antipruritic
Libritabs (chlordiazepoxide)	Antianxiety agent, anticonvulsant, sedative/ hypnotic—controlled substance, Schedule IV
Librium (chlordiazepoxide)	Antianxiety agent, anti-convulsant, sedative/hypnotic—controlled substance, Schedule IV
lidocaine	Ventricular antiarrhythmic, local anesthetic
Lidoject (lidocaine)	Ventricular antiarrhythmic, local anesthetic
LidoPen Auto-Injector (lidocaine)	Ventricular antiarrhythmic, local anesthetic
Lipoxide (chlordiazepoxide)	Antianxiety agent, anticonvulsant, sedative/hypnotic—controlled substance, Schedule IV
Lithane (lithium)	Antimanic, antipsychotic
lithium	Antimanic, antipsychotic
Lithobid (lithium)	Antimanic, antipsychotic
Lithonate (lithium)	Antimanic, antipsychotic
Lithotabs (lithium)	Antimanic, antipsychotic
Loniten (minoxidil)	Antihypertensive
Loraz (lorazepam)	Antianxiety agent, sedative/hypnotic—controlled substance, Schedule IV
lorazepam	Antianxiety agent, sedative/hypnotic—controlled substance, Schedule IV
Lopressor (metoprolol)	Antihypertensive
Ludiomil (maprotiline)	Antidepressant
Luminal (phenobarbital)	Anticonvulsant, sedative/hypnotic—controlled substance, Schedule IV
mannitol	Diuretic

---

* Drug names beginning with a capital letter are trade; drug names beginning with a lowercase letter are generic.

Drug Name	Therapeutic Classification(s)
maprotiline	Antidepressant
Marplan (isocarboxazid)	Antidepressant
Mazepine (carbamazepine)	Anticonvulsant, analgesic
Mebaral (mephobarbital)	Anticonvulsant—controlled substance, Schedule IV
Medihaler-Epi (epinephrine bitartrate)	Bronchodilator, vasopressor, cardiac stimulant, local anesthetic adjunct, topical antihemorrhagic, antiglaucoma agent
Mediquell (dextromethorphan)	Non-narcotic antitussive
Medrol (methylprednisolone)	Anti-inflammatory, immunosuppressant
Mellaril-S (thioridazine)	Antipsychotic
Mentaban (mephobarbital)	Anticonvulsant—controlled substance, Schedule IV
meperidine	Analgesic—controlled substance, Schedule II
mephenytoin	Anticonvulsant
mephobarbital	Anticonvulsant—controlled substance, Schedule IV
meprobamate	Antianxiety agent—controlled substance, Schedule IV
Meprospan (meprobamate)	Antianxiety agent—controlled substance, Schedule IV
Mesantoin (mephenytoin)	Anticonvulsant
mesoridazine	Antipsychotic
Metaprel (metaproterenol)	Bronchodilator
metaproterenol	Bronchodilator
methadone	Analgesic, narcotic detoxification adjunct—controlled substance, Schedule II
Methadose (methadone)	Analgesic, narcotic detoxification adjunct—controlled substance, Schedule II
methotrimeprazine	Sedative, analgesic agent, antipruritic

* Drug names beginning with a capital letter are trade; drug names beginning with a lowercase letter are generic.

Drug Name	Therapeutic Classification(s)
methsuximide	Anticonvulsant
methyclothiazide	Diuretic, antihypertensive
methyldopa	Antihypertensive
methylphenidate	CNS stimulant—controlled substance, Schedule II
methylprednisolone	Anti-inflammatory
methyprylon	Sedative/hypnotic—controlled substance, Schedule III
metoprolol	Antihypertensive
mexiletine	Ventricular antiarrhythmic
Mexitil (mexiletine)	Ventricular antiarrhythmic
Micronase (glyburide)	Antidiabetic
Micro Nefrin (epinephrine hydrochloride)	Bronchodilator, vasopressor, cardiac stimulant, local anesthetic adjunct, topical antihemorrhagic, antiglaucoma agent
Milontin (phensuximide)	Anticonvulsant
Miltown (meprobamate)	Antianxiety agent—controlled substance, Schedule IV
Minipress (prazosin)	Antihypertensive
minoxidil	Antihypertensive
morphine	Analgesic—controlled substance, Schedule II
MS Contin (morphine)	Analgesic—controlled substance, Schedule II
Myidone (primidone)	Anticonvulsant
Mysoline (primidone)	Anticonvulsant
nadolol	Antihypertensive, antianginal
nalbuphine	Analgesic
Nalicaine (lidocaine)	Ventricular antiarrhythmic, local anesthetic
naloxone	Narcotic antagonist
Napamide (disopyramide)	Ventricular/supraventricular antiarrhythmia, atrial antitachyarrhythmic
Narcan (naloxone)	Narcotic antagonist

---

* Drug names beginning with a capital letter are trade; drug names beginning with a lowercase letter are generic.

Drug Name	Therapeutic Classification(s)
Nardil (phenelzine)	Antidepressant
Navane (thiothixene)	Antipsychotic
Nembutal (pentobarbital)	Anticonvulsant, sedative/hypnotic—controlled substance, Schedule II; suppositories under Schedule III
Nervine Nighttime Sleep-Aid (diphenhydramine)	Antihistamine, antiemetic and antivertigo agent, antitussive, sedative/hypnotic, topical anesthetic
Neuramate (meprobamate)	Antianxiety agent—controlled substance, Schedule IV
Neurate (meprobamate)	Antianxiety agent—controlled substance, Schedule IV
nifedipine	Antianginal
Niong (nitroglycerin [oral])	Antianginal, vasodilator
Nitro-bid (nitroglycerin [oral])	Antianginal, vasodilator
Nitrobid (nitroglycerin [topical])	Antianginal, vasodilator
Nitrocap (nitroglycerin [oral])	Antianginal, vasodilator
Nitrocap T.D. (nitroglycerin [oral])	Antianginal, vasodilator
nitroglycerin (oral)	Antianginal, vasodilator
nitroglycerin (sublingual)	Antianginal, vasodilator
nitroglycerin (topical)	Antianginal, vasodilator
Nitroglyn (nitroglycerin [oral])	Antianginal, vasodilator
Nitrol (nitroglycerin [topical])	Antianginal, vasodilator
Nitrolin (nitroglycerin [oral])	Antianginal, vasodilator
Nitronet (nitroglycerin [oral])	Antianginal, vasodilator

---

* Drug names beginning with a capital letter are trade; drug names beginning with a lowercase letter are generic.

Drug Name	**Therapeutic Classification(s)**
Nitrong (nitroglycerin [oral])	Antianginal, vasodilator
Nitrong (nitroglycerin [topical])	Antianginal, vasodilator
Nitropress (nitroprusside)	Antihypertensive
Nitroprusside	Antihypertensive
Nitrospan (nitroglycerin [oral])	Antianginal, vasodilator
Nitrostat (nitroglycerin [sublingual])	Antianginal, vasodilator
Nitrostat (nitroglycerin [topical])	Antianginal, vasodilator
Nitrostat SR (nitroglycerin [oral])	Antianginal, vasodilator
Noctec (chloral hydrate)	Sedative/hypnotic—controlled substance, Schedule IV
Noludar (methyprylon)	Sedative/hypnotic—controlled substance, Schedule III
Noradryl (diphenhydramine)	Antihistamine, antiemetic and antivertigo agent, antitussive, sedative/hypnotic, topical anesthetic
Nordryl (diphenhydramine)	Antihistamine, antiemetic and antivertigo agent, antitussive, sedative/hypnotic, topical anesthetic
Normodyne (labetalol)	Antihypertensive
Norpace (disopyramide)	Ventricular and supraventricular antiarrhythmic, atrial antitachyarrhythmic
Norpace CR (disopyramide)	Ventricular and supraventricular antiarrhythmic, atrial antitachyarrhythmic
Norpramin (desipramine)	Antidepressant, antianxiety agent
nortriptyline	Antidepressant

23

---

* Drug names beginning with a capital letter are trade; drug names beginning with a lowercase letter are generic.

Drug Name	Therapeutic Classification(s)
Novochlorhydrate (chloral hydrate)	Sedative/hypnotic—controlled substance, Schedule IV
Novolin (insulin [regular])	Antidiabetic agent
NTG (nitroglycerin [oral])	Antianginal, vasodilator
Nubain (nalbuphine)	Analgesic
Numorphan (oxymorphone)	Analgesic—controlled substance, Schedule II
Nytol with DPH (diphenhydramine)	Antihistamine, antiemetic and antivertigo agent, antitussive, sedative/hypnotic, topical anesthetic
Omnipen (ampicillin)	Antibiotic
Oramide (tolbutamide)	Antidiabetic agent
Oretic (hydrochlorothiazide)	Diuretic, antihypertensive
Orinase (tolbutamide)	Antidiabetic agent
Ormazine (chlorpromazine)	Antipsychotic, antiemetic
Osmitrol (mannitol)	Diuretic
oxazepam	Antianxiety, sedative/hypnotic—controlled substance, Schedule IV
oxtriphylline	Bronchodilator
oxymorphone	Analgesic—controlled substance, Schedule II
oxytocin	Oxytocic
Pamelor (nortriptyline)	Antidepressant
Panwarfin (warfarin)	Anticoagulant
Parlodel (bromocriptine)	Antiparkinsonian agent
Parnate (tranylcypromine)	Antidepressant
Paxipam (halazepam)	Antianxiety agent—controlled substance, Schedule IV
Pedia Care (dextromethorphan)	Non-narcotic antitussive
pentazocine	Analgesic—controlled substance, Schedule IV
pentobarbital	Anticonvulsant, sedative/hypnotic—controlled substance,

* Drug names beginning with a capital letter are trade; drug names beginning with a lowercase letter are generic.

Drug Name	Therapeutic Classification(s)
	Schedule II; suppositories under Schedule III
perphenazine	Antipsychotic, antiemetic
Persantine (dipyridamole)	Coronary vasodilator, platelet aggregation inhibitor
Pertofrane (desipramine)	Antidepressant, antianxiety agent
Pertussin 8 Hour Cough Formula (dextromethorphan)	Non-narcotic antitussive
phenelzine	Antidepressant
phenobarbital	Anticonvulsant, sedative/hypnotic—controlled substance, Schedule IV
phensuximide	Anticonvulsant
phenytoin	Anticonvulsant, antiarrhythmic
Phyllocontin (aminophylline)	Bronchodilator
physostigmine	Antimuscarinic
pindolol	Antihypertensive
Pitocin (oxytocin)	Oxytocic
Placidyl (ethchlorvynol)	Sedative/hypnotic—controlled substance, Schedule IV
Polycillin (ampicillin)	Antibiotic
Polymox (amoxicillin)	Antibiotic
Pork Regular lletin II (insulin [regular])	Antidiabetic agent
pralidoxime	Anticholinesterase inhibitor
prazepam	Antianxiety agent—controlled substance, Schedule IV
prazosin	Antihypertensive
Primatene Mist Solution (epinephrine)	Bronchodilator, vasopressor, cardiac stimulant, local anesthetic adjunct, topical antihemorrhagic, antiglaucoma agent
Primatene Mist Suspension	Bronchodilator, vasopressor, cardiac stimulant, local anesthetic

23

---

* Drug names beginning with a capital letter are trade; drug names beginning with a lowercase letter are generic.

Drug Name	Therapeutic Classification(s)
(epinephrine bitartrate)	adjunct, topical antihemorrhagic, antiglaucoma agent
primidone	Anticonvulsant
Principen (ampicillin)	Antibiotic
procainamide	Ventricular and supraventricular antiarrhythmic, atrial antitachyarrhythmic
Procan SR (procainamide)	Ventricular and supraventricular antiarrhythmic, atrial antitachyarrhythmic
Procardia (nifedipine)	Antianginal
prochlorperazine	Antipsychotic, antiemetic, antianxiety agent
Profene (propoxyphene)	Analgesic—controlled substance, Schedule IV
Proglycem (diazoxide)	Antihypertensive
promazine	Antipsychotic, antiemetic, analgesic—controlled substance, Schedule IV
Promine (procainamide)	Ventricular and supraventricular antiarrhythmic, atrial antitachyarrhythmic
Pronestyl (procainamide)	Ventricular and supraventricular antiarrhythmic, atrial antitachyarrhythmic
Pronestyl-SR (procainamide)	Ventricular and supraventricular antiarrhythmic, atrial antitachyarrhythmic
propoxyphene	Analgesic—controlled substance, Schedule IV
propranolol	Antihypertensive, antianginal, antiarrhythmic
Protopam (pralidoxime)	Anticholinesterase inhibitor
protriptyline	Antidepressant
Proventil (albuterol)	Bronchodilator
Proventil Syrup (albuterol)	Bronchodilator

* Drug names beginning with a capital letter are trade; drug names beginning with a lowercase letter are generic.

Drug Name	Therapeutic Classification(s)
Prozine (promazine)	Antipsychotic, antiemetic, analgesic—controlled substance, Schedule IV
Purodigin (digitoxin)	Antiarrhythmic agent, inotropic agent
Pyopen (carbenicillin)	Antibiotic
Pyridamole (dipyridamole)	Coronary vasodilator, platelet aggregation inhibitor
Quinidex (quinidine sulfate)	Ventricular and supraventricular antiarrhythmic, atrial antiarrhythmic
quinidine	Ventricular and supraventricular antiarrhythmic, atrial antiarrhythmic
Quinora (quinidine)	Ventricular and supraventricular antiarrhythmic, atrial antiarrhythmic
Razepam (temazepam)	Sedative/hypnotic—controlled substance, Schedule IV
Regular Iletin I (insulin [regular])	Antidiabetic agent
Regular Iletin II (insulin [regular])	Antidiabetic agent
Regular Pork Insulin (insulin [regular])	Antidiabetic agent
Reposans-10 (chlordiazepoxide)	Antianxiety agent, anticonvulsant, sedative/hypnotic—controlled substance, Schedule IV
reserpine	Antihypertensive, antipsychotic
Restoril (temazepam)	Sedative/hypnotic—controlled substance, Schedule IV
Ritalin (methylphenidate)	CNS stimulant—controlled substance, Schedule II
Ritalin SR (methylphenidate)	CNS stimulant—controlled substance, Schedule II
Rivotril (clonazepam)	Anticonvulsant—controlled substance, Schedule IV

* Drug names beginning with a capital letter are trade; drug names beginning with a lowercase letter are generic.

Drug Name	Therapeutic Classification(s)
RMS (morphine)	Analgesic—controlled substance, Schedule II
Roxanol (morphine)	Analgesic—controlled substance, Schedule II
S-2 Inhalant (epinephrine hydrochloride)	Bronchodilator, vasopressor, cardiac stimulant, local anesthetic adjunct, topical antihemorrhagic, antiglaucoma agent
Sarisol No. 2 (butabarbital)	Sedative/hypnotic—controlled substance, Schedule III
Seconal (secobarbital)	Sedative/hypnotic, anticonvulsant—controlled substance, Schedule II; suppositories are under Schedule III
secobarbital	Sedative/hypnotic, anticonvulsant—controlled substance, Schedule II; suppositories are under Schedule III
Sectral (acebutolol)	Antihypertensive, antiarrhythmic
Sedabamate (meprobamate)	Antianxiety agent—controlled substance, Schedule IV
Serax (oxazepam)	Antianxiety, sedative/hypnotic—controlled substance, Schedule IV
Sereen (chlordiazepoxide)	Antianxiety agent, anticonvulsant, sedative/hypnotic—controlled substance, Schedule IV
Serentil (mesoridazine)	Antipsychotic
Serpalan (reserpine)	Antihypertensive, antipsychotic
Serpasil (reserpine)	Antihypertensive, antipsychotic
Sertan (primidone)	Anticonvulsant
Sinequan (doxepin)	Antidepressant
Sintocinon (oxytocin)	Oxytocic
SK-Tolbutamide (tolbutamide)	Antidiabetic agent
Sleep-Eze 3 (diphenhydramine)	Antihistamine, antiemetic and antivertigo agent, antitussive,

* Drug names beginning with a capital letter are trade; drug names beginning with a lowercase letter are generic.

Drug Name	Therapeutic Classification(s)
	sedative/hypnotic, topical anesthetic
Slo-bid (theophylline)	Bronchodilator
Slo-Phyllin (theophylline)	Bronchodilator
Sofarin (warfarin)	Anticoagulant
Solfoton (phenobarbital)	Anticonvulsant, sedative/hypnotic—controlled substance, Schedule IV
Solu-Medrol (methylprednisolone)	Anti-inflammatory, immunosuppressant
Sominex 2 (diphenhydramine)	Antihistamine, antiemetic and antivertigo agent, antitussive, sedative/hypnotic, topical anesthetic
Somophyllin-T (theophylline)	Bronchodilator
Somophyllin (aminophylline)	Bronchodilator
Sparine (promazine)	Antipsychotic, antiemetic, analgesic—controlled substance, Schedule IV
Spectrobid (bacampicillin)	Antibiotic
spironolactone	Antihypertensive, diuretic
St. Joseph for Children (dextromethorphan)	Non-narcotic antitussive
Stadol (butorphanol)	Narcotic agonist-antagonist, opioid partial agonist
Stelazine (trifluoperazine)	Antipsychotic, antiemetic
streptokinase	Thrombolytic
Sucrets Cough Control Formula (dextromethorphan)	Non-narcotic antitussive
Sus-Phrine (epinephrine)	Bronchodilator, vasopressor, cardiac stimulant, local anesthetic adjunct, topical antihemorrhagic, antiglaucoma agent
Sustaire (theophylline)	Bronchodilator
Talwin-NX (pentazocine)	Analagesic—controlled substance,

23

Drug Name	Therapeutic Classification(s)
	Schedule IV
Tambocor (flecainide)	Ventricular antiarrhythmic
Taractan (chlorprothixene)	Antipsychotic
Tavist (clemastine)	Antihistamine
Tavist-1 (clemastine)	Antihistamine
Tegretol (carbamazepine)	Anticonvulsant, analgesic
temazepam	Sedative/hypnotic—controlled substance, Schedule IV
Tempra (acetaminophen)	Non-narcotic analgesic, antipyretic
Tenormin (atenolol)	Antihypertensive, antianginal
Tensilon (edrophonium)	Antiarrhythmic, cholinergic agonist
terbutaline	Bronchodilator
Thalitone (chlorthalidone)	Diuretic, antihypertensive
Theo-24 (theophylline)	Bronchodilator
Theo-Dur (theophylline)	Bronchodilator
Theobid (theophylline)	Bronchodilator
Theoclear (theophylline)	Bronchodilator
Theophyl (theophylline)	Bronchodilator
theophylline	Bronchodilator
Theospan-SR (theophylline)	Bronchodilator
Theovent (theophylline)	Bronchodilator
thioridazine	Antipsychotic
thiothixene	Antipsychotic
Thorazine (chlorpromazine)	Antipsychotic, antiemetic
Thor-Prom (chlorpromazine)	Antipsychotic, antiemetic
timolol	Antihypertensive, antiglaucoma agent
Timoptic (timolol)	Antihypertensive, antiglaucoma agent
Tindal (acetophenazine)	Antipsychotic
tocainide	Ventricular antiarrhythmic
tolazamide	Antidiabetic agent

---

* Drug names beginning with a capital letter are trade; drug names beginning with a lowercase letter are generic.

Drug Name	**Therapeutic Classification(s)**
tolbutamide	Antidiabetic agent
Tolinase (tolazamide)	Antidiabetic agent
Tonocard (tocainide)	Ventricular antiarrhythmic
Tornalate (bitolterol)	Bronchodilator
Trancot (meprobamate)	Antianxiety agent—controlled substance, Schedule IV
Trandate (labetalol)	Antihypertensive
Tranxene-SD (clorazepate)	Antianxiety agent, anticonvulsant, sedative/hypnotic—controlled substance, Schedule IV
Tranxene-SD Half Strength (clorazepate)	Antianxiety agent, anticonvulsant, sedative/hypnotic—controlled substance, Schedule IV
tranylcypromine	Antidepressant
triazolam	Sedative/hypnotic—controlled substance, Schedule III
Tridione (trimethadione)	Anticonvulsant
trifluoperazine	Antipsychotic, antiemetic
Trilafon (perphenazine)	Antipsychotic, antiemetic
trimethadione	Anticonvulsant
Trimox (amoxicillin)	Antibiotic
Triptil (protriptyline)	Antidepressant
Truphyllin (aminophylline)	Bronchodilator
Tusstat (diphenhydramine)	Antihistamine, antiemetic and antivertigo agent, antitussive, sedative/hypnotic, topical anesthetic
Twilite (diphenhydramine)	Antihistamine, antiemetic and antivertigo agent
Tylenol (acetaminophen)	Nonarcotic analgesic, antipyretic
Uniphyl (theophylline)	Bronchodilator
Utimox (amoxicillin)	Antibiotic
Valadol (acetaminophen)	Nonarcotic analgesic, antipyretic
Valdrene (diphenhydramine)	Antihistamine, antiemetic and antivertigo agent, antitussive,

23

---

* Drug names beginning with a capital letter are trade; drug names beginning with a lowercase letter are generic.

Drug Name	Therapeutic Classification(s)
	sedative/hypnotic, topical anesthetic
Valium (diazepam)	Antianxiety agent, skeletal muscle relaxant, amnesic agent, anticonvulsant, sedative/hypnotic
Valorin (acetaminophen)	Nonarcotic analgesic, antipyretic
valproic acid	Anticonvulsant
Valrelease (diazepam)	Antianxiety agent, skeletal muscle relaxant, amnesic agent, anticonvulsant, sedative/hypnotic
Vanceriase (beclomethasone)	Anti-inflammatory, antiasthmatic
Vanceril (beclomethasone)	Anti-inflammatory, antiasthmatic
Vaponefrin (epinephrine hydrochloride)	Bronchodilator, vasopressor, cardiac stimulant, local anesthetic adjunct, topical antihemorrhagic, antiglaucoma agent
Velosef (cephradine)	Antibiotic
Velosulin (insulin [regular])	Antidiabetic agent
Velosulin Human (insulin [regular])	Antidiabetic agent
Ventolin (albuterol)	Bronchodilator
Ventolin Syrup (albuterol)	Bronchodilator
verapamil	Antianginal, antihypertensive, antiarrhythmic
Viscous (lidocaine)	Ventricular antiarrhythmic, local anesthetic
Visken (pindolol)	Antihypertensive
Vistaril (hydroxyzine)	Antianxiety agent, sedative
Vivactil (protriptyline)	Antidepressant
warfarin	Anticoagulant
Wymox (amoxicillin)	Antibiotic
Wytensin (guanabenz)	Antihypertensive
Xanax (alprazolam)	Antianxiety agent—controlled substance, Schedule IV

* Drug names beginning with a capital letter are trade; drug names beginning with a lowercase letter are generic.

Drug Name	Therapeutic Classification(s)
Xylocaine (lidocaine)	Ventricular antiarrhythmic, local anesthetic
Zarontin (ethosuximide)	Anticonvulsant
Zepine (reserpine)	Antihypertensive, antipsychotic

---

* Drug names beginning with a capital letter are trade; drug names beginning with a lowercase letter are generic.

Bibliography

American Heart Association: Textbook of Advanced Cardiac Life Support. American Heart Association, Dallas, 1994.

American Heart Association: Pediatric Advanced Life Support, American Heart Association, American Academy of Pediatrics, Dallas, 1994.

Beck, RK: Pharmacology for Prehospital Emergency Care, ed 2. FA Davis, Philadelphia, 1994.

Brown, KR and Jacobson, S: Mastering Dysrhythmias: A Problem-Solving Guide. FA Davis, Philadelphia, 1988.

Deglin, JH and Vallerand, AH: Davis's Drug Guide for Nurses, ed 4. FA Davis, Philadelphia, 1995.

Hudak CM, et al: Critical Nursing: A Holistic Approach, ed 6. JB Lippincott, Company, Philadelphia, 1994.

Jones, SA, et al: Advanced Emergency Care for Paramedic Practice. JB Lippincott Company, Philadelphia, 1992.

Physicians' Desk Reference, ed. 49. Medical Economics, Montvale, NJ, 1995.

Sanders: Mosby's Paramedic Textbook. Mosby Lifeline, St. Louis, 1994.

Thomas, CL (ed): Taber's Cyclopedic Medical Dictionary, ed 17. FA Davis, Philadelphia, 1993.

Vallerand, AH and Deglin, JH: Drug Guide for Critical Care and Emergency Nursing. FA Davis, Philadelphia, 1991.

Notes

Notes

Index

Numbers followed by an "f" indicate figures; numbers followed by a "t" indicate tables. More common drugs are listed on pages 80 through 107.